twicks twicks out twice

The Successful Recovery of a Stroke Survivor

To Sarah and Iain
with very best wishes
Richard

twicks twicks out twice
The Successful Recovery of a Stroke Survivor

Published by: Able Publishing

ISBN: 1 903607 76 0

978 1 903607 76 3

www.ttot.co.uk

Cover design: Nigel Orme
Photography: Richard Denyer
Portrait: Maddy Pikarsky

Typesetting and production:
Able Publishing
www.ablepublishing.co.uk

Printed in the UK by:
Impress Print, Northampton

To Maddy and Nigel,

and all kind friends

Acknowledgements

A lot of people have helped me with the text of this book and with its preparation for print. If there are any mistakes, they can only be mine. So many thanks — in clear, not squashed into a dense paragraph — to:

Lizzie Barnard
Simon Horton
Mary MacMaster
Jan McAllister
Caroline Roberts
Roger St. Vincent-Pickard
the staff at Able Publishing

and Will Watts without whose spur this work may never have been completed.

Table of Contents

ORGANISATIONS AND INFORMATION SOURCES

PART ONE
THE COMMENTARY

To begin with

After 40 years of full time work, it lost its entertainment value. In 2002 I sold up in London, moved to Norwich and became a part-time student at the Norwich School of Art and Design. The course: MA Photographic Studies. I was half way through year two and was beginning to find a path to follow towards my final project.

On Friday 5th of March 2004 I was in a good mood, looking forward to more School work. About eight o'clock in the evening, I was watching a very old movie on a DVD. Without warning I found myself looking at the world sideways. I was lying on the floor. Furthermore, without any memory of dialling a number — however short — I was talking to the ambulance service about how to find me so that they could take me somewhere safe. It was all a mystery: nausea, sleepiness, inability to understand where I was, but no pain. I had had a stroke.

That's how it started.

The Journal is what I wrote while I was recovering in hospital and during rehabilitation, a contemporary record. It is the second part of this book. This part, the Commentary, is a companion to the Journal, a memoir based on it. It gives the details of my successful recovery and digs around among my thoughts and feelings, and it starts here …

The outside of me

The history

The history starts with that fall in my living room; it continues with three weeks in the Norfolk and Norwich University Hospital (a.k.a. N&N) and then 12 weeks in the Colman Hospital's rehabilitation ward, Caroline House.

The first few minutes

The DVD I was watching that Friday evening was *The Man with a Movie Camera*, (Russian, 1929, silent, fascinating technical achievement by director Dziga Vertov). Without any preliminaries I found myself lying on the floor looking sideways; everything was at right angles to where it ought to have been. A further mystery was that I was on the telephone talking to the ambulance service. Why would I be doing that? I guess I was telling them what was happening. How I fell to the floor I do not know. How I telephoned the ambulance service I don't know either.

With some difficulty I described to the ambulance service where I lived and how to get there. That was about 8:30. It is still a little bit of a surprise to me that I was able to do it. The ambulance people arrived in a few minutes but it took over an hour to get me out; they had to call the police to break down the front door and let them in.

A word about my flat: it was on two floors above a shop. The many-times-altered building was somewhere between 300 and 400 years old, and in my flat there were no right angles, no flat floors and, in the upper staircase, no two steps alike. In fact the upper staircase is more like a Picasso painting of a staircase. The front door to the flat is in a small courtyard accessed by a narrow passage from the street. What I called my living room was on the upper floor.

I can remember moments in the journey down the two flights of stairs. It was difficult because of those stairs. At one moment I know I was sitting in an ambulance chair with a man underneath me; I must have been balanced on his head.

The first few hours

The next thing I remember was being in a hospital, somewhere, throwing up my guts. I was very keen on this activity until a nurse calmed me down; I abandoned my endeavours and fell asleep. (Someone may have given me an arm-full of sedative but I've got no evidence for this.) The hospital was the Norfolk and Norwich University Hospital, N&N for short.

By two o'clock the next day, Saturday, they took me for a brain scan (CT variety) that I don't now remember. I've seen the scan. It is a scary thing to contemplate, even now; have a look. And it left no doubt about the diagnosis: I did have a stroke. And the scan report suggests damage which includes Wernicke's Area, a part of the brain that deals with speech.

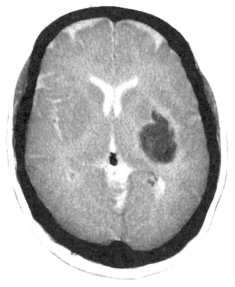

My next vague memory is eating a meal; I was half sitting up, in or on a bed. I remember thinking "They don't know

As the hospital report says: "large acute haemorrhage in left parietal and temporal lobes." It's about the size of a walnut – in its shell.

what's wrong with me but they're feeding me! Is that wise?" In making that analysis I remember also thinking that they were giving me a meal so that they could fulfil some government target. I now know — from reading my hospital notes — that during the weekend my swallowing was tested. I guess that was what was really happening.

The first few days

I was settled into the N&N's Gunthorpe Ward Stroke Unit. The ward had six beds with elderly gentlemen as patients, half of them seriously ill which meant there was a fair amount of ongoing care and attention from nurses.

At the beginning of this experience I asked no questions: it never crossed my mind to find out what ailment I was suffering from, I had no particular fears, I wasn't in pain, I could more or less see straight although there was some disturbance to the vision in my right eye.

I was certainly in hospital — dressed in undersized hospital pyjamas — and I was sitting up and seemingly OK except for this inability to move my right arm and right leg. Indeed the whole of the right hand side of my body was knocked out: no sense and no power.

It was on the day after I was rescued that I received a first visit from my family. Having failed to contact me by phone, in the ordinary way of keeping in touch, my sister and brother-in-law went to my flat to find me. They found the broken front door and straight away searched for me by phoning hospitals.

I was very pleased to see them, and I hope it showed; they certainly seemed pleased to be seeing me. Little did I know how anxious they were, indeed horrified. We exchanged pleasantries and there was plenty of smiling and nodding, and they went away. Only later did I discover, from my sister Maddy, that I was almost completely incoherent. Although my utterances were English words — or neologisms very like English — many of them were in unusual combinations and made little sense, and I used a fair number of obscenities. Maddy told me how she acted the part of a cheerful visitor but was in tears on the way to the lift to leave the hospital, crying "I don't want my brother to be a la-la."

There can be no doubt that — in those first few days — I was somewhat disorientated, confused about what was going on around me and happening to me. Incoherent speech should not have come as a surprise.

Read the first few pages of my Journal. From conversations with my son Roger, my neighbour David W, and several others of my visitors, the writings during the whole of March give a very accurate impression of how I spoke: fast, rambling, gobbledygook, all with an air of that great self confidence which I genuinely felt. I was using an almost random selection of words. They weren't totally random, it was as if I chose them because they meant something similar or sounded similar to what I wanted to say. My hospital notes include the phrase "fluent dysphasia" … a wonderfully appropriate technical description.

The first few weeks

… well two weeks and six days to be exact, I stayed in the N&N.

I recognised that I was very lucky in having so many visitors. Conversation was generally brief and was attended by mutual, though friendly, incomprehension. My visitors' reports are in the later section in this book about my speech and its recovery.

As well as family and friends, I had medical visitors: a very smart consultant in a suit, very sensitive, listening and describing what I had, it was a stroke; he seemed to appear most days. I had other visitors as well but not every day, Dr Jeremy G and Dr Louisa N; they were from Caroline House, part of the Colman Hospital. They had come to have a look at me to see if I would be a suitable case for treatment at their place. I slowly came to understand Caroline House to be a specialist rehabilitation centre for patients who had brain injuries and who could benefit most. Another medical visitor was Senior Nurse Jenny C; I do know she came to tell me things or to ask me things but the details are well beyond my recall.

During the second week in the N&N I was put under pressure by an infection. My remaining strength degraded leading to a complete loss of right-hand-side movement and to a progressive loss of words. After a five-day treatment with antibiotics, speech came back but movement remained weakened.

Maddy and brother-in-law Nigel were particularly helpful and continued to be overwhelmingly so for many weeks to come. They brought me clothing which I could wear – and which I did wear – when I left the N&N and went to Caroline House.

Maddy did a magic thing for me when I was in the N&N: she brought me a wad of photocopier paper and some soft pencils. She said that I could do drawing. The first thing I did was writing; I started a Journal. Even before Maddy had brought me the paper I was making little notes – mostly meaningless – on a tiny little writing pad. My writing was left-handed – something new for me; it improved after I had written several pages. Drawing became part of the Journal, by way of illustration.

At about the same time, Maddy brought me a dictation gadget that I had asked for, so that I could keep some kind of diary. But I couldn't understand how to work it and asked her to take it back. Later, I had other gadgets to learn – or relearn – such as the mobile phone and my telephone bank.

The phone took me a couple of weeks of experimentation just to get the basics right. It took me days more to remember how to work the rest of the phone's features.

Luckily I got the banking sorted out quickly. Mine is a telephone bank and I was worried that I might not be able to get through the security questions. I did the phone call and got the security questions right first time; I think that is because it wasn't language problem in the ordinary sense, it was a well-practised ritual.

When I went to Caroline House I had nothing but my clothes. Maddy and Nigel made several trips to my flat to fetch more clothes and some of the daily essentials of life (shaver, toothbrush etc). Nigel helped me out greatly with some necessary paperwork and we figured out a scheme whereby, between us, we could draw cash and pay bills. Maddy helped me out equally greatly with some necessary purchases, in particular: new underwear and T-shirts, and what I call sloppy trousers.

The season at Caroline House

What is Caroline House?

I went into N&N on a Friday and came out nearly three weeks later on the Thursday and went, wearing my own clothes, to Caroline House. The patients there all have different kinds of brain injury: industrial and traffic accidents as well as strokes.

The house has about three dozen beds — roughly half of them in single-occupancy rooms — plus lounge, restaurant and essential offices (fig. and lit.). It is built all on one level and surrounded by gardens.

I wasn't initially aware of the significance of moving to this particular location; good fortune had certainly attended me! It is a world-class rehabilitation centre with a skilled nursing staff and a comprehensive gathering of specialists in speech, physiotherapy, occupational therapy and psychology. I was always encouraged to do for myself everything that I could. I was never allowed to be lazy; this is not to say I was never allowed to sleep; I *was*. Some nights I did sleep long and very well, as if my whole body, every cell, had filled itself with sleep.

Starting rehabilitation

What a weird experience! To be able to use the left hand side of your body but not the right. And on my right, I would have no idea where my arm was or my leg unless I felt for it with my left side. Even if I did know where my limbs were I couldn't move them. Isn't a leg heavy? But my left hand abilities revealed themselves remarkably quickly. I don't remember explicitly experimenting with writing but I must have done so as a youngster, to see what it was like. Quite soon I was able

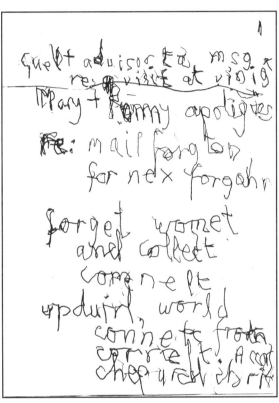

This is (probably) the earliest writing. It looks like a To Do list of four or five items

to write in a fairly neat hand anything that I needed. Writing was slow but accurate enough for posterity.

Sooner than I expected I started on physiotherapy. Each Monday morning a timetable of activities for the week was posted on the inside of my door. It didn't look very much, an hour here and a half-hour there: physio, speech, OT and psychology. But a scheduled hour's physiotherapy might take up only 10 minutes; after a month of doing nothing, the physical effort was beyond anything I could have predicted.

Physio was training in two senses: firstly learning how to move limbs and next practising movements in order to regain strength. My very experienced physiotherapist, Joni C (also my Key Worker and guru), with different assistants on different days, put me through an ever-changing battery of exercises. As my legs became retrained so I could stand for a few moments when transferring to and from the wheelchair. After another few weeks, I could stand long enough to wash myself and brush my teeth.

Standing up straight and tall was a grand sensation I still take a moment to enjoy. And then, with help — *mirabile dictu* — I could take steps. Steps became walking — with a stick: first on the level, then over rough ground in the garden, and lastly up and down stairs. I keep the stick. For many weeks after leaving Caroline House I used it outdoors but indoors only to go to the bathroom in the night. Now I carry it for walking — as a signal of possible unsteadiness — but rarely use it though it does help going up hills.

I had no idea how many muscles had to be attended to in order to be able to do anything at all, never mind coördinated or repeatedly. We spent much of the time on exercises for lower-body strength; upper-body strength comes back on its own because you do it to yourself even when you're in a wheelchair.

There is a lot of overlap between physio- and occupational therapy. OT is more about life skills: washing and dressing, cooking and eating, and handling everyday objects. I've got plenty to say about it later. But physio includes plenty of life skills too: walking over rough ground, changing direction, carrying a small load. And it was in physio that I learned to pick myself up after a fall, with help or without.

Unmatched medical and nursing attention

For several years I have had a well-controlled, minor heart condition. Part of the control was to take Warfarin, a blood thinner. Here's the deal:

- with thinned blood there is a raised risk of stroke from a bleed in the brain;

- without the blood-thinner there is a raised risk of stroke from a clot moving to the brain.

It felt like a very grown up decision that I would have to make: what kind of treatment to accept: to thin or not to thin. I had three or four conversations with the doctors one of whom prepared for me a beautifully written summary of the situation.

It doesn't matter what the decision was, that isn't my point. What I am saying is that the medical staff worked to make sure I really understood the problem. The attention I got from everybody was at this level of care and skill.

At the time we had this teach-in, a new brain scan (MRI variety) was made that showed "… improvements from the bleed (like a bruise getting better)." A nice extra from the doctors: that they were willing to give me the details, and in plain language too.

Material evidence of the continuing care and attention which so impressed me takes the form of very full medical notes. Practitioners all added their notes in an English-and-code mixture so that all knew what the others were discovering and deciding.

My visitors

Visitors always cheered me up. Some came frequently and some just once or twice. Penny W and Mary M came every couple of weeks and brought a breath of normal air, chatting about their ongoing experience of Art School, and news of people we knew. They always skilfully judged the right length of a visit, never too long. Neighbours David W and Mrs W came several times with genuine inquiry after my condition plus reports on the state of my flat — as seen from the outside — and the goings-on of other neighbours. And Lizzie B brought me the most impressive bunch of flowers, grand in style and long living in the vase. I feel rude not to list everyone who came to see me but you know who you are!

Family came often and in different combinations, for a quick Hallo or for an extended get-together. They brought me treats: home made eatables and my favourite chocolate biscuits.

On one visit, my niece Flossie brought a hanging bird feeder which she had made for me. She set it up on the branch of a tree just outside my east-facing window. I looked forward to a scene from Nature's show but, sadly, the birds hadn't been to RADA and wouldn't act.

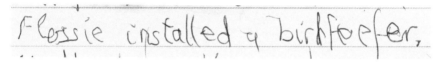

From Journal, 11 April

The other patients

We patients came together daily for lunch and tea. We arrived by three routes: pushed in a wheelchair, self-propelled in a wheelchair and walking. Not every one of us came for every meal. We settled into more or less regular groups, three or four to a table, changing as patients went home or new ones came.

The degree of mutual support among patients was a bonus from which we all drew. The encouragement may have been a tad formulaic but it was certainly well meant. We appreciated each other's success; I remember a round of applause going up the first time Michael walked unaided into the restaurant and another when I did the same. I'm choking up as I recall these moments.

We rather liked that rarity: a joke. At one lunch I was sharing a table with three other men one of whom was permanently morose and had no conversation. I felt my upwardly and backwardly extending forehead and said, only to myself "My hair has slipped down the back of my head." I'm still not quite sure why I said it or why it was funny; two men laughed and my usually silent neighbour grinned out loud.

Patients also had a weekly "fun hour" organised by assistants. I found these difficult to begin with for two reasons. The first was because of the too-fast flow of conversation (more about that later) and the second was that I sometimes got flustered in a crowd when I had become the centre of attention.

Changing rooms

Single rooms

When I first came to Caroline House I was put in a room near to the nurses' station. Such patients as those who may need a lot of attention are generally placed there when they arrive.

After hardly a fortnight I was moved to room 33. This was both good news and bad news: as the Journal points out (8 April). Good news: it was light and airy, lots of window-glass and views over the garden in two directions. Bad news: I finished up with noisy neighbours. There were two types: the ones to leave their telly on so loud you can hear it till 1:00 in the morning, and the ones who have a noisy family visiting in order to have a row. Whenever I had visitors, I closed the door to give us the privacy we prefer and to reduce any annoyance to others. (Is that too much to ask? in a hospital?)

My next-door neighbour and I easily negotiated the sound levels. The one further up the corridor could not or would not turn the sound down or close his door … hmm.

Several weeks further on I was moved to "The Flat." The Flat is a bed-sitter where patients can practise being at home. It has a small kitchen, an excellent *en suite* bathroom and a cosy little sitting-room which is also the bedroom. I enjoyed the privacy and relished the opportunity to be independent.

I liked it there although I have to say it was very tiring for the first few days. I was walking about much more and "working hard" at tough jobs like making my own breakfast and, some days, my own supper too. I was beginning to appreciate that when I left rehab, my biggest undertaking would be daily living.

Lost in the shower

A stage in my recovery came when I was well able to walk to and fro.

One morning I went for my shower and, at a point when fully soaped, the light went out. It's like this: the separate lavatory and shower room were served by lights switched by a single switch. Someone had come out of the lavatory and switched all the lights off together. There I was, in the dark, covered in soap and laughing.

Luckily for me my balance was good enough; I was able to rinse off and search with my hands for a towel without falling over. I completed my ablutions and got enough of a bathrobe and towels around me to get back to my room.

Apparently, I learned, euphoria is common in new stroke survivors. It certainly heightened my feeling of amusement at being artificially blinded for those few minutes.

Going home

The general idea of The Flat is that patients go home from there; this was the original plan for me. But I wasn't quite ready to go home when another patient came to the flat and I was bumped. I moved across the corridor to a different room for the remainder of my stay at Caroline House.

In a manner of speaking I wasn't going home; I was going away. After all, living in my own wonky-floored, crazy-staired, multi-storied flat was not on the cards. I was going to a well-equipped rented flat but one with no personal possessions in it. "Going home" from Caroline House was generally done in stages: a one-night sleep-over, a weekend and a permanent move. The schedule for each stage being judged by the success of the previous. For my one-night stand, I made a list of the things I would use if I were at home; there were 30 items, from food in the fridge to spare socks; and Maddy and Nigel fetched them for me from the old flat.

The sleep-over was a success and so was the weekend. Indeed the weekend was such a success that there was effectively no break before I moved permanently. Maddy and Nigel filled my fridge and freezer so that I could get my bearings without the immediate need to go shopping.

As I was actually moving, permanently, the whole family gathered (the next weekend) to pack and transport everything personal that converted "a" rented furnished flat into "my" rented furnished flat. They did a full day's removal work in a morning and, I must say, a good job it was.

I still haven't got all my books and pictures or the bits of furniture I can fit in. At the moment that's OK; there are still signs of life in the old flat for when it goes on the market.

By good fortune, I was made — and I accepted — the offer of a 3-wheeled electric buggy, the "Scoota", at a friendly price. My forecast for myself came true in a big way: that my biggest undertaking would be daily living. I was whacked just getting through the day. For the first three weeks, I don't remember going out. I'm sure I did otherwise all my coffee would have been black and my Shredded Wheats dry. The buggy is a boon, I treat it like a short-distance car: drive to where you want to be then get out and walk. For a long time, walks were uniquely within supermarkets and the hall of my old flat (to collect the mail). I also went back fortnightly to Caroline House as a visitor to have lunch and greet everyone I knew.

As the months have followed so walks have taken on a new significance: exercise. I frequently walk round the block, Saturdays I go for the paper and, when visiting folks, I can be persuaded to stroll a bit. I am sure this will build up eventually to the point where walking will be for any distance I choose.

Mutual admiration

All the time I was in Caroline House I had great respect for every individual member of staff. Each, in their own style, prodded me and prompted me to make progress. And, as far as I could, I accepted their guidance and followed their instructions. It was their care and encouragement which inspired me to work so hard and take pride in my progress.

I found it embarrassing that *they* took inspiration from *me*. Surely, I was doing what anyone else would do in my situation. Alas, it seems not ... what it does seem, I learned, is that some patients remain stolidly in bed or wheelchair "waiting to get better."

So far, I have been writing about what happened by way of a history; the Journal fills in with lots of details. What follows now is a more specific and detailed look at my physical and mental recovery.

Physical recovery

Progress towards recovery and the eventual degree of recovery are different for every stroke survivor. There is no doubt that — even though my stroke was described as severe — my recovery has been remarkable in both speed and outcome.

Through all the years of my career I have been a journal writer and a note keeper. Every time I went abroad to work in a new location I would make a generous record of my impressions, more a travelogue than a diary and almost as good as photographs. In the later years, as a technical author, I had properly to understand what I was writing about, analyse it, and re-express appropriately for its audience.

The Journal is by way of being a continuation of my record-keeping obsession; the Commentary my analysis. You are part of a very mixed audience; let's all hope the expression is appropriate.

In this section I will describe much that I originally wrote in the Journal but, now, I will try to give more insight and write separately about different aspects of physical and mental progress.

On the physical side of my recovery, sensation returned — but slowly, and not completely — and the power of movement increased week by week, thanks mostly to the physiotherapists. By the time my 15 weeks were over I was strong enough to be released into the wild and live on my own again (plus an NHS walking stick and the above-mentioned electric buggy).

What is a stroke?

Please take what comes next as the impressions of a survivor … I am not a doctor. A stroke is a brain injury. If it comes with little or no premonition, it's called acute. It comes in two varieties: a bleed from a broken blood vessel inside the brain, and a clot in a blood vessel which blocks it.

Whether from flood or drought, a portion of the brain is damaged. Permanent damage is part of the story but there is also the equivalent of a surrounding bruising which fades with the passing of time. Different people have offered me different timescales for recovery: 18 months for most of the recovery, and three, five, 10 and even 15 years for the rest.

As well as the stroke damaging some nerves permanently, it temporarily disconnects nerves by a swelling. It is the reconnection of nerves that underlies recovery. Some reconnection comes about among existing circuits in the brain as the pressure from the bruising lifts. I am convinced brand new connections are made as well and old connections used for new purposes.

There are differences in the survival rates and recovery rates for the two types of stroke; don't ask me for details, ask a specialist.

In all this, the rest of the body is undamaged. Parts of the body are made unserviceable because they are not getting their normal exercise, from the nervous system being out of touch with itself.

What could I do for myself

I was in the N&N for three weeks but I remember very little of the regime, how much was physically handled by nurses and how much I could do for myself. I know I could use the urine bottle, I could feed myself, I could jiggle about in a chair. But I couldn't get in or out of bed unaided or change my pyjamas or wash. Every action was slow and tiring.

As the rehab weeks progressed, the combination of physiotherapy, occupational therapy and my own hard work, took effect. Thus most of these homely actions came back so that by the time I went "home" I could manage every essential part of living. The range of extra activities will build slowly.

Sensitivities

Hand and foot

After all these months, I still go to bed hoping that in the night the feeling in my right hand will come back completely. It doesn't of course but it has improved.

To allow for the deficiency, I am adapting either myself or the world around me. I have certainly adapted my behaviour in the matter of avoiding hot things by testing temperature with my normally sensitive, left hand. I adapted my camera — thanks to Nigel for the idea — by sticking a bit of "hard" Velcro on the release button. The button now has a rough texture and it stands proud a millimetre or so.

With the passing of time more and more actions become automatic or at least easy. For example I am winning more battles with my shirt-cuff buttons while standing up rather than after being forced to sit down (to rest).

Feeling in the limbs

Even after months my right leg didn't gain any skill in knowing — when in bed — where it was. It could be hanging out and dangling on the floor getting cold and I would never know until I tried to move or turn over. Why "was"? It is still true, sometimes, and still a surprise.

The movement of the margin

When I say "margin", I mean the vertical equator, that imaginary line running down the centre of the body. That line demarked the left hand side which could feel and do anything, and the right-hand side which was initially powerless. My guess is that while the two halves of the body have distinct nerve networks there is surely a bit of overlap at the centre line.

This idea of a margin was most noticeable on my head. As the margin wandered, over the weeks, from the centre towards the right, so the corner of my eye, my nostrils and the back of my head all itched, at different times and in different degrees.

The sense of touch to the right of the margin improved rather slowly; but it did improve. For example I remember the day when my elbow and my ribs first felt each other … a magic moment!

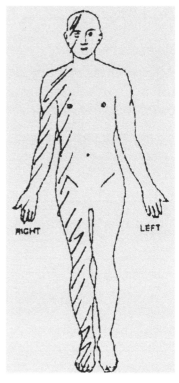

The loss of feeling as recorded at the N&N

Eyesight

There was, initially, quite a disturbance to the sight in my right eye (see Journal, A5 Notebook page 3). It resolved itself gradually and completely within five weeks. That kind of disturbance goes by the poetic name *homonymous hemianopia*.

Like the other physical symptoms it was nothing to do with the affected part — in this case the eye — it was an effect of the brain injury.

Left   Right

ok on testing but reports is not there.

Homonymous Hemianopia? ☑

Assessment by opthalmoligist? ☐

Assessment by optician? ☐

Comments
need to assess further

The early N&N evaluation of my short-lived vision problem.
See Journal, A5 Notebook page 3, for my own evaluation

Hearing

My hearing on the right had become, and has remained, slightly less sensitive. It is sufficiently less sensitive sometimes to disturb conversation, for example in those noisy places such as a cafe or restaurant where one would like to focus one's hearing. I talk about this in more detail in the next chapter, in the section on speech.

Temperature, reactions to stimuli

Sensitivity to temperature is very reduced; water from a tap always feels cold unless it is too hot. I burned myself more than once on the hand or wrist while cooking before I learned to approach pots and pans with my left hand to check their temperature. (I have had some interesting lessons taken from observing the way in which the skin heals; the body is a marvellous machine.)

The physiotherapists at Caroline House take on second-year students for four-week spells of practical training. The students also prepare a short lecture which they present to staff. My physio, Joni, invited me to hear the presentation by the student who had had me as a victim (ahem, ahem, I mean client). Her topic concerned the workings of the nervous system. Let's remember that there was nothing wrong with my limbs or their nerves, only something wrong with their connections inside my head. The lecture included a description of how the nerves that connect to temperature and to pain travel a shared path and can get mixed up. Joni later asked me if we could test the situation in my case. Sure enough anything hot on my hand hurt like a drawing pin in the forearm; iced water likewise. It was a case of "Ow ow that's my arm" instead of "My goodness, that's a cold hand."

Hot body, cold body

This may be all about weather-sensitivity or it may be all about what happens to someone who spends a lot of time in bed. Even in the warmest weather I felt I needed extra layers on the bed when going to sleep for the night. Then other times, regardless of the weather, I would need to take all the layers off. This apparently trivial question is not one that I have resolved.

Nerve pain

My paresthesia – nerve pain – is the constant background of unpleasant sensation in parts of the right side of my body. It can be so unpleasant that it is genuinely painful; some patients really suffer and have to follow a pain management regime.

I am one of the lucky ones; it's there all the time but it isn't everywhere and it doesn't distract. So where? and what? Mainly under the skin of the extremities on the right hand side: forearm, hand, ear (the external parts), lower leg, ankle and foot. If I keep still, I don't notice anything; if I move about, or touch or work with the hand or foot, it always appears. Description is difficult. For me, nerve pain is like a combination of pins and needles, a scald and the left-overs of a slap. If my leg got tired after walking too much, the sense of ache was taken over by an increase in that paresthesia.

Accidents

In the N&N there wasn't much scope for accidents but I was found sitting on the floor one time. It was because I had overbalanced and slid off my chair while reaching – ever impulsive – for something on the bedside table.

While my subsequent rehab progress was good, it wasn't always as good as I thought it was. This continually lead me to attempt more than I was truly capable of. The result was a number of falls. Sorry to say I once bruised some ribs and another time cracked one.

Evening time in The Flat was when I had the worst falls. Just when I was standing up to get ready for bed. Having spent an hour or so sitting and relaxing at the end of the day, I would stand up without taking care to look at my feet to see where they were going. Left foot good, right foot bad … totally unaware of where it was. I fell over because the foot was not where I imagined it to be, so "Ow ow! "

After I left Caroline House I had a fun fall in my new flat. Squatting under the desk, I was plugging cables for the computer. When I finished, I got up. No I didn't, I fell over in a gentle, quite elegant backward roll. So I thought "OK, now I'm here I'll have a five minutes break." No ribs this time, just private embarrassment.

Weight

At the beginning of March I weighed 13 stone 5 pounds (85 Kg); by the middle of April I was down to 12 stone 3 pounds (78 Kg). For me this was good news. Over many months previously I had been aware that I was eating too much in the evening. This was a left-over habit from my working years when the eating pattern was sandwich-and-soda lunch and heavy supper. I was trying to implement a new plan: sensible lunch and a light supper. As a result of this weight loss after the stroke I more comfortably fitted my trousers and, so far, in the months which have followed, I have stayed the same.

Pacing oneself

I found it easy to do too much. When I was feeling energetic I would exercise more and stay awake longer. After a day or two being so active I would collapse in a heap, almost unable to move. Joni changed my programme: a rest after lunch every day … that did help. But from then until now I haven't got the hang of knowing when I'm going to be tired; I only know when I am tired.

I have given myself some help in this regard, most especially since I came home, by way of a morning "ritual." Getting up, breakfasting, tidying the kitchen and such domestic necessities, I start and finish between eight and 10:30. Some days they will be done before 10 o'clock! By way of this ritual, I am already pacing myself through the first half of the day. At this stage I will already know if I'm too tired to be "busy." If I'm feeling energetic I would attend to a shopping trip, more writing as I'm doing at this moment or — as with any household — sorting out essential paperwork, again!

Before the stroke, getting out and walking used to be an integral part of every day: short shopping trips, to and from Art School, and promenading by the river. A shopping trip — using the electric buggy as transport — is a fair substitute for a walk. Typically, in the afternoon I will sit and read, or just sit.

The best advice I have received on the subject came from a brochure, one of a big collection of charity, social service and health service brochures and leaflets that — I guess — every brain injury patient is offered; here it is:

> Recovery is usually a slow process, and you may find it easier to cope if you try to follow the advice below:
>
> - Make sure you get adequate rest. It is quite normal to feel very tired in the months following a stroke.
>
> - Try to take each day as it comes. You may find that it helps to set yourself small and realistic goals to work towards, such as putting on your shoes yourself or walking a short distance (if you are mobile).
>
> - Make sure you do things at your own speed, even if this seems unbearably slow both to you and others. Setting yourself a time limit will simply increase your feelings of frustration. It is important to build up confidence in what you can do and to accept this takes time.
>
> - Try to keep to a regular routine and look for ways in which you can revive old interests or take up new

ones. An occupational therapist may be able to make suggestions and offer practical advice.

From *After your stroke: a first guide*,
The Stroke Information Service, by kind permission.

When I first read this advice it rang true straight away; months later it still does and I have wholeheartedly passed it on to other stroke survivors. As my own recovery has progressed — with periods of overdoing things — I can assure you that the advice is sound.

Physiotherapy recovery

As occupational therapy, so physiotherapy covers a lot a subjects. I think of physio as the exercise yard where I was trained and tested for strength and stamina, and "tricks."

Exercises

Each week I had a schedule of activities including physio sessions. Some of the sessions were exercises, following a programme. These were jolly hard work but increasingly strengthened my legs and back.

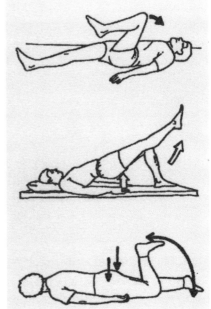

Work on my upper body was less concentrated; daily living worked on that. Try putting on a tee shirt with one of your arms "playing dead. " You'll be amazed at how much strength it takes and how just a little improvement makes the job much easier.

A small selection of the apparently mild but actually strenuous exercises. (Copyright © Physio Tools Ltd.)

Walking

The main topic on the retraining list was walking. The very first attempt had me upright and attended by the physiotherapist and — I am sure — three assistants. They were variously holding me upright and monitoring my balance and the positions of my feet. And as I attempted each step they gave me instruction and encouragement. Oh dear! The flow of information was too fast, coming from what seemed like a dozen voices. I felt quite queasy after a few steps and gave up! We agreed that next time I would hear just one voice however many assistants were surrounding me.

Over the weeks, walking progressed from a handful of paces with a quad stick (a walking stick with four feet) to strolls round the grounds over grass and garden paths, up and down kerbs, and up and down stairs.

I matured with a lazy right foot which tended to scrape the ground unless I took particular care. Over the months since leaving rehab, this foot has come more-or-less into line with its partner and my gait is only slightly uneven.

Everyday tricks

What do I mean by "everyday trick"? I mean ordinary actions like putting the shopping away, and getting things off the top shelf or the bottom shelf when you need them. And "tricks" includes recovering from minor accidents such as picking things up after you've dropped them and stepping round a spill of coffee in the kitchen. Picking things up includes picking yourself up if you fall.

I spoke before about the cross-over between OT and physio. Training in this variety of actions came as part of the latter. I had several sessions playing tricks and games designed to give confidence and practice in these unobvious, everyday activities.

Balance

Part of physiotherapy is assessment of the patient; among several indexes of performance was the Berg Balance test. In my case it gave the most impressive measure of the power of physiotherapy, and a result which — I'm sure — could not have been gained any other way.

This balance test is a sequence of some dozen or so tasks involving sitting and standing, looking around while sitting and standing, reaching out in front, turning round on the spot ... all different and increasingly difficult. What did I score? After four weeks, 17/56, after eight weeks, 44/56 and after 11 weeks 52/56.

The "blinded in the shower room" incident was right at the end of that period, thank goodness!

Occupational therapy, recovery

Like physiotherapy, OT took plenty of effort. It was directed towards doing the ordinary activities which anyone would expect to be able to do.

More than merely moving and strengthening body and limbs, I was learning to coördinate them for doing all my simple jobs. There was a continual interplay between strength and dexterity; as each improved, so the other could be worked on.

Write a sentence with a verb and a noun below

~ I eat the bread

From the Reading & Writing part of a neurological screening test. This was done in an OT session on the first Monday at Caroline House.

I've several times mentioned that there is overlap between physio- and occupational therapy. In an early physio session, I was instructed to turn the pages of a glossy magazine with my right hand, left hand strictly behind my back, while standing at a lectern. I struggled to get a finger under the front cover of the magazine or to slide the cover over from the first page. After several finger-aching and wrist-aching manoeuvres I got the magazine open. I acted the eager magazine reader by going through the contents list, aloud. (Not all of it obviously, there's always far too much.) Then I started work on the first inside page. More pointless fingering. Suddenly a brainwave: "Is it alright if I lick my finger?" I asked "Oh yes" they said, giggling and laughing (*and you know who you are*). It was then I realised I didn't have the strength to raise my fingers to my face … I had to lower my head to the desk. I admit that we all had a good laugh; they had foreseen my difficulty whereas I hadn't appreciated how weak I was. I did turn the page.

Even though I developed some fingertip sensitivity, it took a very long time to build strength that I could use for the most trivial of skills.

Ongoing training

My "OT" Jessica D had me playing all kinds of games: picking things up and putting them down, throwing and catching, feeling for objects hidden in a bucketful of rice, judging the weight of objects, putting on and taking off nuts and bolts. I lost several games of plastic boule! but did fairly well at reaching and grabbing the bowls wherever Jessica held them in space around me.

A good trick she taught me was to use a mirror technique to train myself to carry out ordinary actions. The trick is to do the action with the stronger hand and imitate it, as if in a mirror, with the weaker. That's how I got back to brushing my teeth manually (instead of electrically) and eating with a spoon (yes … it's difficult). I used the mirror method when I learned by imitation to curl my toes momentarily when pulling on my jeans, to avoid getting them trapped in the stitching of the hem.

During the weeks which followed the start of my training, I practised and worked to be able to do such simple things as: putting my watch on, tying my laces or, in the first place, scratching the back of my neck. Every little advance such as these made the day a red letter day and I recorded them in my Journal.

I developed exercises and skills out of class as well as in. Initially shoe-lace tying was a great trial … I failed for quite a long time but it came to me in a while. I did children's wooden jigsaw puzzles as the basis for developing dexterity and stamina. Getting the pieces turned the right way round and picking them off the floor after flicking them there by accident, both of these were muscle-building exercises that came free with every piece.

Mechanical aids

Different people among my therapists offered me different kinds of mechanical aid. I started my mobility training with the wheelchair and continued it with sticks … no objection there. But I could not see myself using bent-handle forks and spoons at meal times, or kitchen gadgets for the one handed. Pen grippers to help with writing didn't please me either. This refusal was partly to avoid the mere appearance of being disabled and dependent, and partly because I felt it was the only way to reach my target: being normal. If I seemed ungrateful, I'm sorry. But lucky me to have had the choice.

During my continued recovery at home I have developed the techniques of — among others — doing up my own shirt buttons and locking the back door "on auto." Next target? Using chopsticks!

OT for shopping and cooking

A small addition to the Caroline House range of diet took the form of meals patients cooked for themselves. Part of the occupational therapy work was to do shopping and cooking, and I did this half a dozen times in the weeks towards the end of my stay. You can see the list "meals what I cooked" at the end of the Journal.

Shopping was exciting! Really. It was a great event: to get out of Caroline House a couple of times and go to Waitrose. At the early stage I was in the wheelchair all the time. For the second visit I was in the wheelchair till we got to the sales floor, then I walked with a stick.

To begin with, when I was cooking, my hands were too greatly mismatched in strength to be able to work together; I had several lessons in technique. One of the meals I made — I always think I invented it — is "Cowboy's Breakfast": baked beans on grilled bacon on toast. When I cooked this for my lunch, the beans part was easy, the toast part was easy, the grilled bacon was a bit fiddly but it worked out. When it came to eating there was a new problem: my hands had been so busy, cooking, that they were barely strong enough to cut up my bacon. Lesson: if you have weak hands, cut your bacon into little pieces with scissors before you cook it (or eat it with scissors).

How good it was to be able to do more and more as the 15 weeks progressed. And how grateful I am for the therapies to which I was treated. As great as any of this was my recovery of speech and writing.

The inside of me

In the last section, I concentrated on the external person: myself as a case, a stroke survivor getting physically back to normal. Now I want to tell the story of the inner man: the one who communicates by speaking and listening, by reading and writing, and who has thoughts and emotions.

Speech, capabilities and recovery

All the time I was in the N&N my family came to visit me: my sister Maddy and brother-in-law Nigel, who live locally, and my son Roger who visited Norwich for some of that time. On each occasion I was happy to see them and they were happy to see me, smiling and nodding as before. I was convinced that we were having an ordinary conversation, following normal give-and-take rules. In fact most of my share was gibberish, it was made up of words — quickly grabbed from my mind's store — that might sound or mean something similar to the words I intended. In those early days, my tone of voice appeared to match the sense of what I believed I was expressing: sometimes cheery, other times serious and at all times confident. It didn't occur to me that there was any problem or that they were having any worries about my condition.

Other friends came to visit me during that time: Penny W, Mary M, Richard D and Lizzie B — fellow students and staff from the Norwich School of Art & Design — and my old neighbour David W with Mrs W. I later asked them about the quality of my conversation during that period; they all confirm the family's story. I asked them to write me their recollections of how I was during the first few days and weeks.

Here are extracts from their e-mails to me/about me; this is part of what my fellow student Mary M said:

> The first time we came, just a couple of days after your admission to hospital, you appeared, unsurprisingly, quite stunned. I remember you saying, very politely even in your rather sad state, that if we had asked you would have preferred not to see us until a later date. We stayed only a few minutes and communication was limited to a few short sentences and holding your hand. Speech was clearly very difficult and your mouth seemed partly frozen; ... and you were obviously pretty unhappy.
>
> The next time, perhaps a week or so later, although still seriously affected, you had cheered up enormously, wearing your own clothes and propped up in bed. For a while speech remained quite slurred and sometimes difficult to understand; retrieval of vocabulary often an effort – occasionally even frequent use words escaped you but you never seemed to mind, that's just how it was and you seemed very accepting about getting us to fill the gaps. If it existed, you didn't allow any frustration to show. Gradually over the weeks speech became easier to understand and you took more interest in the outside world. One day you were excited about beginning to write and as use of your arm returned you were able to explain improvements. Then when you moved to Caroline House, especially when you took up residence in the flat, you seemed suddenly almost back to normal – there was the day you could stand, then walk......! I think that speech improvement was in parallel but I can't remember that very exactly; I think we usually forgot you had had problems at all.

Lizzie B, another fellow student who came to see me in the N&N, reported to me, in part:

> In some ways he was better than I expected and in some ways worse. There was no movement whatsoever in the right side of his body and if he wanted to move his right

hand he had to pick it up with his left and put it where he wanted it to be. It also meant that he could not write in his normal way.

... the consequences of the stroke seemed to have affected his cerebration, his speech and his ability to write. There were moments of intense clarity of thought and speech followed by patches of finding it difficult to articulate words and phrases, or even marshal the expression of ideas, as though the part of the brain which formulates concepts and develop themes was blocked. The best analogy I can think of is an oiled up spark plug – so the engine was firing on only three cylinders.

At some point, it may have been at our second meeting, probably ten days to a fortnight after his stroke, Richard showed me some notes he had been making describing what he was thinking or what had been happening to him. The notes were incomprehensible. It wasn't just that he was writing with his left hand, the marks did not always resemble letters in the English alphabet and therefore did not make recognisable words.

The comforting thing about the notes (why did I need comforting? He was the one with the problem!) was that Richard himself knew it was gobbledegook. So that made it alright.

Weeks later, after Richard had left hospital and moved to Caroline House he showed me some new writing he had done. By this time he had mastered writing with his left hand and his brain was better able to co-ordinate ideas. This time the notes did make sense.

Lizzie is right about not making recognisable words but I think the penmanship was acceptable. That was rather like my speech: fairly clearly enunciated but not very meaningful.

And, also from my time as an MA student at NSAD, the course leader, Richard D, came within the first week and had this report for me:

> ... Not sure exactly, but I think between 4 – 6 days. You were of course talking nonsense, so it was difficult initially to determine to what extent the stroke had had any affect whatsoever. But seriously though ... You were clearly only too happy to converse, so the problem was wrestling with the memory of articulate pre-stroke Richard and trying to reconcile this up with gibbering post-stroke Richard. Mostly this didn't work, so we're left with much nodding and gesticulating and the hope that we haven't communicated anything that might add to your problems.
>
> In a slightly bizarre way, I am envious of your (temporary) altered state, and I wonder what it must feel like to be you at this moment. What is nice is that if you are apologising because you know you cannot be understood, then we can't hear that either, so it is a dialogue without the need of many normal social graces, and is therefore strangely liberating when you get into the swing of it.
>
> On subsequent visits communication becomes clearer and normal service is gradually resumed, complete with social conventions. I try consciously to make your condition not the sole topic of conversation – it threatens to bore us both – and at least we have photography / Art School stuff to talk about too.

Over the first week or two I continued to believe in my own clarity of speech and logic of conversation. But it was clear to everybody else that I had lost control over my mouth. As the first few weeks progressed, I started to recognise that I was making mistakes and began correcting them more and more often. A reading of my Journal, which started before the move, shows clearly how my speech capability, matched by my writing, improved. Indeed, the quality of the writing was revolutionised in a period of just three days as March turned into April.

I do know that my early speech was not entirely incoherent. I remember explaining to one of the staff that I did <u>not</u> want a television that worked, I wanted them to turn it off. On another occasion, at night, I contrived to have a very noisily spoken nurse sent to another ward because my sleep was so disturbed.

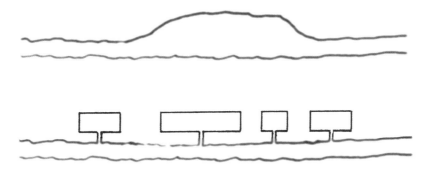

My visualisation one night of the extremes of reactions: to easily tolerated soft-focus quiet speech and the painful hard-edged noisy.

During the first couple or three weeks after the move to Caroline House I repeatedly asked the nurses to let me know if I was being offensive. They always said that they didn't take any notice (and, so, my question was never answered).

Aphasia

Lost words

Plenty of times I couldn't find the word for what I wanted to say. At the beginning this was a severe problem; every sentence — if not every phrase — had a word I couldn't find.

A trick of speech which I developed early on was to experiment out loud with a word that I was aiming for. If the word didn't come to me straight away I would mutter trial words increasingly quietly, testing them to see if they fitted. When I found the word (or something like it) that seemed right, I would speak up again. I used this trick both with the family and with the therapists and nurses; I guess it was about six weeks before that one faded.

The N&N Speech and Language Therapist used this mixture of words and symbols to describe my early habit when I would mutter experimentally. A possible plain language interpretation is: "word-finding difficulties along with decreased volume of speech accompanied by apparent jargon."

As I say, to me, speech was not a problem. Even though I was aware of its inaccuracies I could feel a change from week to week which encouraged me to think that that part of my life would be normal soon enough.

Lost souls

Apart from a non-specific difficulty in recalling some words, that difficulty which I overcame by experimenting *sotto voce* with words which might be right, apart from that I had a problem with names.

Whenever I met a new member of staff I asked them their name. I would forget that name within 10 seconds and either ask again or, later, try to read their badge or ask someone else what the other person's name was. (I noticed that staff did not introduce themselves.)

It had always been a point of pride in me that I could learn and remember people's names; there's no word people love hearing more than their own name!

This difficulty persisted for many weeks. It was not until near the end of my stay that learning and remembering started to come back to me, and it has now stayed.

Speed limit

In the early times I did have difficulty in understanding what was being said to me. If someone spoke too fast or if two or more people spoke at the same time I would have a real problem understanding what was happening.

A good example of this was in the ordering of my meals for the next day. I settled down to a standard breakfast but lunch and supper were different all the time. Whoever was filling in the chart would read off the main courses and vegetables so fast that I could not take in the information. Here is a typical main-course menu offering:

Spoken as

Roast chicken and stuffing, vegetable and bean cottage pie, minced chicken and stuffing, or flaked fish portugaise? With roast potatoes, creamed potato, peas or carrots?

Heard as

Roast chicken and *fast-talk-fast-talk-fast-talk-lots-of-words-all-too-fast-I'm-not-getting-this-can't-understand-all-this-oh-oh-dear* or carrots?

I asked them to read each item and leave a good gap before the next so that I could understand and visualise what each item was.

For the same reason, I didn't watch TV for weeks; I found the flow of information too fast to cope with. News broadcasts foxed me within minutes and I found "entertainment" too loud and too complicated. This difficulty has pretty well gone away but I still get disconnected and isolated by some things that never bothered me in the old days: fast speech, yes; but also speech in noisy surroundings and speech in an accent I'm not used to, for example: the American drama series *West Wing* on TV. I used to be able easily to follow the stories acted out with their underplayed, faux-natural dialogue. Now the combination of fast and sometimes mumbled speech has me foxed again and I switch on the subtitles to help me out. Whereas formerly I could understand speakers with strong regional accents, now they too often give me a problem.

At the beginning of this section, *The inside of me*, I included some quotations from friends' e-mails. They vividly describe my speech in the earliest days. These days those same friends tell me I am "just as you used to be" and I thank them for saying it, and I believe it.

Speaking and listening have pretty well come under control. Apart from minor lapses in talking and hearing (I am 65 after all) I think I am "normal." Writing follows a similar story.

Writing

For much of my career I did technical writing; I produced several millions of words in specifications, "how to" manuals, briefing papers, standards and magazine articles. In this section I want to go into the questions of what happened to my writing abilities and how well they have recovered.

Within a few days of moving to Caroline House, I was writing normal, proper English text. My speech was still subject to error and my listening subject to incomprehension. Within a couple more weeks — subject to some aphasia (names and word lists) which has now mostly gone away — everything came more or less clear again.

During my recovery, two major milestones passed with respect to handwriting. The first was recovering the ability to write using my right hand. Even though my left-hand writing was acceptable it felt good to come home. The second — on my PC at home — was to use Dragon NaturallySpeaking dictation software; it is a most impressive tool with a high degree of accuracy, and it saves handache.

When I was first in hospital, my sister offered me a dictation machine. I thought and said that I would not be able to work it, it was — at that time — too complicated. Now, I wish I had mastered it; it would have provided a fascinating record.

When she brought me paper and pencils with the suggestion of doing drawing, my record-keeping compulsion took over … I had to write. It seemed to me the most natural of endeavours and I proceeded with it enthusiastically and totally unselfconsciously. And it does provide a fascinating record.

Writing the Journal

Hand-writing: left and right

It is still a bit of a surprise that my left-handed writing was so clear so soon. At the start, I knew that I was writing slowly; part of the struggle was that I was sitting up in bed without any easy-to-use rest for the paper. At the start, the meaning of what I wrote was largely hidden. In spite of the awkwardness of the process of doing writing, I used the space on the pieces of paper to organise the material into sentences. and paragraphs

Three months later, I noticed that I had put my watch on "on auto"; previously a tiresome task needing much concentration. I was so intrigued by this observation that I decided to try writing with my right hand. See the Journal for 31 May when, suddenly, right-handed writing appears all at once.

Typography

Initially, while I was making my notes and lists I had no realisation that the text itself made no sense; but I was aware of the "typography". I used indented lists and paragraphs to lay the material out, and commas, full stops and capital letters for sentences, and even semicolons, all as well as writing the jargon text that — I believed — made sense.

Drawing

It is interesting that something of the drawing side of me stayed in quite good shape; I had been to life drawing classes some years before. When I was doing a little sketch — the dancing girl — I was aware that it was at least as good as any sketch I'd ever made for a similar purpose, and at two levels: rather pleased I was doing it with my left hand, and rather pleased I was getting such a good result. I had created the sketch using many short, wispy strokes. (See Journal, A4 sheet 1.)

Also good progress on all fronts esp. RH which is both stronger and cleverer so that, for example, cooking on Thursday was a lot easier and this morning I put my watch on without noticing.

Also good progress on all fronts esp. RH which is both stronger and cleverer so that, for example, cooking on Thursday was a lot easier and this morning I put my watch on without noticing, and then I tried writing — seems to be OK!

The repeated paragraphs which demonstrated that I had successfully returned to right-hand writing. The right is wobbly but serviceable.

Whendney 23 (o … ie 3rd of 3rd follow dasigh).

1. Charyth: the right rightfly right-on sole you and
   improgafal   if improv axemadoylay.
   Aolay on on but a vere is is is is
   stregthen and a latactact & roughnnenneining

2. These right row raironmess-
   — Chowraisp, partitral 1 + 2 thurmail & 5 load film

   — Chaim   OK to to pail up nurnes (noses only)

   — Chaim clasesy to a glean new grenny to
   from from to from (from very weark why read)

Transcribing manuscript to typescript is enough to show the accuracy
with which the original layout was controlled in terms of both indentation
and line spacing (and is indeed a style I had earlier chosen).

Absence of obscenities in writing

In the first few weeks, when I was in the N&N, I'm told that I used a fair quantity of obscenities in conversation. The writing at that time — and for a week or two after — is near-impossible to interpret but even with an imaginative reading there are no obscenities to be found. If there were none in the writing, perhaps I wasn't speaking any to the extent that I feared.

Errors detected while writing and while reading later

In the earliest days I was using a trick of experimenting with words, more and more quietly, till I found the one I wanted (so I thought). Look at the Journal; right there is the evidence that I used this trick when writing; have a look through A4 sheets 1, 3 and 7. See the trial spellings of words, see the trial placements of apostrophes. Journal for 28 March contains a good example with four goes at spelling and punctuating the same word.

As with speech, so with writing: I quite soon started detecting errors and correcting them. You can see what I mean by looking at the shape of the graph here: It covers the period from when "proper" English text starts to the end of the Journal.

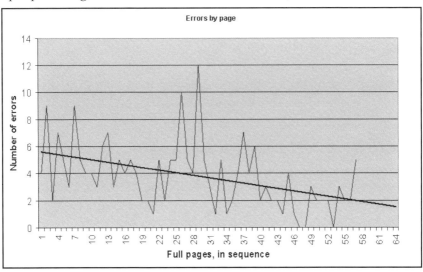

I counted the number of errors on each page; the analyst at work again. See how the number goes down as the pages turn. The heavy line smoothes out the results and shows the number of errors per page reducing from almost six to fewer than two. That peak around pages 26 to 30 came when extended Journal entries were spread over two days; no wonder there were a few extra mistakes. How my hand must have been aching.

I distinctly remember the parallel between my speech corrections and my writing corrections. Writing left handed (about which more later) was for me a fairly slow process. So I could have a word in mind, start writing it, then — because I was writing so slowly — forget what the word was and write something else. I soon got into the habit of reading my Journal most carefully to see that I had the word that I wanted. There remained many errors in the Journal, some of which I fixed up later.

There are interesting distinctions between error-detection while speaking and while writing. First of all, when speaking, we all make minor errors — slips — in speech and when we correct them "on the fly" no-one pays them any attention. With handwriting, the errors are more noticeable, even when they are corrected. Also with writing, you can go back days, weeks or centuries later and re-read the material. I did indeed re-read my Journal weeks later and made further corrections then. Corrections made at the time are fairly obvious because there are crossings out on the same line as the rest of the writing; corrections made later are above or below. Unfortunately there is no sure way, now, of distinguishing the two different kinds: contemporary or later on.

We are human, we communicate; we are human, we think and feel. I've gone through speaking and writing in the last two sections; I've put my thoughts about the latter in a separate section, next.

Intellect

Introspection is sometimes down-played as a method of research. The analyses that follow are based on my introspection so a pinch of salt may sometimes be appropriate.

My early observations

I observed myself making an early judgement on hospital procedure when I had a thought that I mentioned earlier: "They don't know what's wrong with me but they're feeding me! Is that wise?" (and thinking it was so that they could fulfil some government target). This was based on a false interpretation: they were testing me for being able to swallow. Even so, I did observe something and was able to make a judgement even if faulty; as well as being a judgement on clinical procedure, it was political.

As a quaint example of a specific capability left untouched: even in the first days after the stroke, I could tell the time correctly, out loud and without hesitation.

While on antibiotics, during the second week in the N&N I felt my vocabulary declining. Any time during my internal monologue when I lit upon a word and considered its meaning, that word would disappear from my vocabulary. That was a real worry and I thought my brainpower must be declining. But then as the 5-day course of antibiotics finished that part of my wits came back.

Their early observations

The multi-disciplinary notes from both N&N and Caroline House contain many descriptions of my state of mind and of my thinking ability. By the middle of April I could score well in The Cognitive Assessment of Minnesota, that was very reassuring. After that the notes described my aphasia, memory problems and moods rather than the straight thinking skills.

Doing arithmetic

I had good training in maths, and in arithmetic as part of maths. My father was an engineer and schooled me in the meaning of numbers, their weights and significances. With him, I learned to do fast, approximate calculations in my head and — most important for an engineer — how to get the decimal point in the right place. And I enjoyed and pursued the study of mathematics at school and university.

Since the stroke, I have lost my sharpness in that skill; it's slowed down a lot and I'm better now using paper and pencil. A significant but not a crucial loss.

Keeping up with the plot

Earlier I described how fast, accented speech gave me difficulties, but that's not the whole story. I did also have trouble with the stories. Recognising who is who, what is happening, the significance of clues, all these passed me by for a while. I can say, these months later, that following the plot is much, much less of a difficulty though, like doing arithmetic, I have slowed down a bit.

Misunderstanding anatomy

Without repeating the details I have to tell you that I did have some troublesome times with the workings of my innards. (You may come across the page in the Journal which sets out my thoughts on this subject.)

I really was in two minds about what was happening inside me. My logic told me how all the bits inside connect up (to the limits of my knowledge of anatomy). In the first weeks, with all those delirious thoughts, my fancy was that many of the bits did not connect at all.

It was indeed a clear couple of months before these difficulties disappeared and my innards started working in a "regular" way.

Sleep patterns

From the beginning right up to the present day I have had a mixture of sleep patterns. They tell me this is normal but it is the extremes of pattern that I find quite remarkable. Some evenings I feel really dozy and go to bed early and sleep for 12 hours. Other evenings I feel dozy, go to bed and stay awake till one or two in the morning. Some days I wake up easily, other days I stay immobile till the middle of the morning.

In the early days these long sleeps left me next to unconscious even when I woke up. It was a time when I felt that each long sleep led to a mini-recovery in some part of my body, my senses or my understanding.

More recently I find the erratic patterning to be more an irritation than a marvel. It seems to change — without notice, without apparent cause — every few weeks.

Dreams

In the early weeks I had the most vivid and complicated dreams. The dreams were in colour, they were frequently populated by people whom I knew and they seemed to be very long dreams.

One of the most vivid was a rerun of the movie *Sunset Boulevard* inside my head. It was in the first couple of weeks of arriving at Caroline House and as I watched the movie in my dream I realised that I could select scenes and replay them, going backwards or forwards through the whole of the movie. (Do you remember the last scene: "I'm ready for my close-up. Mr DeMille."?)

As the complexity of the dreams abated so "storylines" became clearer. I can't tell you what these lines were because they went out of my head as soon as I woke up. But I knew they were there and I was continually interested in what was going to happen next. I think in many of these dreams I must have been much nearer to waking than sleeping because I was conscious of having made quite difficult, complicated calculations and decisions.

Emotions

Earliest responses

My son Roger has told me that I expressed, very clearly, suicidal thoughts along the lines of "If I don't come through this I will top myself." It is not a stream of thought that flowed for very long; it dried and was replaced by my ambition, my hunger for recovery "… to be as normal as I used to be." Indeed, Roger tells me, I seemed almost suddenly to be treating my recovery as a new, interesting project to undertake.

Roger wasn't the only one to note my mood over the first few days. Visitor Mary M had come only two or three days after the stroke and said that "… you were obviously pretty unhappy."

Most of the time after the first couple of weeks at Caroline House my emotional tone settled and, I felt, was very positive. Certainly I worked hard in all my classes and was able to turn many of them into games. I always enjoyed company; it was in my lonely times that I felt less confident and less hopeful.

Ups and downs

For family and friends I put on a cheerful face; it was — in any case — truly a joy to have visitors. But at certain moments, often for two or three days at a time, I would be very low. These patches of tear-stained misery came on in the lonely moments, the evenings. Several times I was overwhelmed by the hugs and encouragement of the nurses. They really believed I would get better and they made me believe it too. I was so lucky to be looked after by the

Caroline House nurses and I love them all; they had such a calming influence on me when I got into a tizzy about my inadequacies and the slowness of my progress.

I can't say that these blue moods had any particular cause unless it was the idea that I might never get better or that I might always be dependent. It was certainly that last thought that my OT Jessica had written in her notes on me, that "Richard became tearful and reported it was due to him gaining some insight into the level of his difficulties + implications on his care." The psychologist made a similar report. (That was in the my first full week at Caroline House.)

Looking back from almost a year later I can say that I have got over those early fears. My ups and downs now are more physical than emotional.

My space

In the past I've never had problems with making speeches or addressing an audience, and I still don't. In the past I never had problems with being in crowded places, but now I do. The weekly social hour at Caroline House I found awkward because everyone in that small crowd was too near, and I was expected to "perform" — under pressure as I saw it.

I have had the same feeling in shops when I'm examining something or talking to sales staff and some other shopper gets too close. That feeling of my space being invaded is entirely new. This point may seem too trivial to mention but I do so to point out that peculiar side effects arose after the stroke, the kind of effects you wouldn't expect.

Lost and found

I did have one fortnight of miseries which had a very specific cause: the time I lost my early Journal. The A4 pages were in a soft plastic folder. The folder went missing. It contained the earliest and most precious of my writings. I asked everyone if they could help me find it, and everyone did help me but it didn't turn up. I feared that it may have been thrown away by accident — by me or by someone else. I was made cross by the idea that maybe someone had seen it and ignored it, as a piece of children's work not worth keeping, and had thrown it out with the Sunday papers.

My bad temper lasted a week and more. But, joy of joys, we found the folder, and misery and anger receded. (See Journal, 11 April.) I can feel, with hindsight, much easier going about losing the writings. How our memories can treat us kindly as distant memories become sketchier.

Attitude changes

Self-propelled change from patient to convalescent

At about Week 8 of my stay in rehab, my way of thinking about myself changed. I stopped being a patient and started being a convalescent. I gave myself permission to be much more self-sufficient: instead of being cosseted I started to do much more for myself. For the nurses this could be quite boring, like when watching me battle to get a T-shirt on or off or — later — struggle with my own socks and shoes.

Personality changes

Approaching this question is rather like approaching a lottery winner with the question: "Will these millions change your life?" However people might try to convince you otherwise the answer is still "Yes."

So it is with a stroke. Obviously there are physical limitations to what you can do; many of these limitations — for me — are going away. Since leaving Caroline House I have been living on my own quite successfully. The changes in my inner life are more significant.

As a generalisation I can say that I am a softer person; more aware of the world and much more accepting of the world as it is, and sensitive to the troubles of others and the difficulties they face. This generalisation is certainly true in respect of my relationships with other people. I am more easily moved to tears than I ever was before.

But this is 2004 with all its troubles in the wider world and I am as cross as anybody about the extreme and negative results of politicians' decisions, and the way they spin those results and decisions.

What happened next

The making of this book has taken over a year and a half. It's taken this long for several reasons. As life has held surprises and interest in areas other than telling this story, so I have been diverted a lot of the time. Also — as I have often said — it is easy to do too much; I would lose a couple of days or even a fortnight recovering my energy after overextending myself. Some of the time I could do nothing more than daily living.

The transcription of the Journal, and the writing and editing of the Commentary were done mostly during the first few months of my recovery. Writing now, as the final editing and proofing come to completion, and at the second anniversary of the stroke, I can say more about the successful recovery.

The outside recovery

The outside of me has continued to make progress; in many respects I can already say that I lead a normal life. It is dexterity which has led the way; strength and stamina are still catching up.

What follows is a week-by-week summary of the steps in getting somewhere back to normal. When I made this list, I was quite taken aback with the numbers of steps that came in some of the shorter periods. The biggest changes came in weeks seven to 10 — when I was probably at my moodiest — and in the last four weeks in rehabilitation. At those times, progress seemed impossibly slow. Obviously I wasn't understanding what the side-effects of stroke really meant for me. Looking back, I can only marvel at what actually happened.

It hasn't been all sunshine. The lack of clear sensation in my leg and foot means that when walking the placement of my feet for the next pace can be a few centimetres off; enough to make me a bit drunken-looking.

Paresthesia has stuck around; Any tiredness in a right-side limb becomes quite pronounced. I'll say this again: "Every case is different."

Week by week

This is the tally of what more I could do in each of these weeks:

1 Sitting unaided, feeding self; right side out of action.

3 (end of week) Start using wheelchair (at Caroline House), powering and steering with left foot.

5 Transfers (to and from bed, w/chair etc) require only one helper instead of two.
   Standing (with care) for Wash & Dress.
   Dressing self (but not shoes & socks).
   Able to lift arm to scratch neck (my first big "magic moment").

6 Controlled movement — flexing and tapping — in right foot.

7 Start learning to walk (with rails and with quad stick).
   Sudden increase in finger skills (eg during dressing and OT "games").
   Beginning of light-touch sensitivity in right limbs.
   Right-eye vision finally clears after previous continuous improvement.
   Transfers to and from w/chair without help, but supervised.
   And much, much more!

11 All daily activities unsupervised after the first few days in The Flat.
Wheelchair no longer used around Caroline House or the rest of Colman Hospital.

15 Capable of going home alone, and doing so.

20 More independence; working hard at shopping.

30 All errands much easier (shopping, collecting mail from old flat) using buggy.

50 Walk a mile once a week and walk half a mile twice a week. Often leave walking stick at home.

100 Continuing stamina improvement. Resting less during the day. Can walk up to a mile or mile-and-a-quarter, on up to three times a week. Rarely take walking stick out.

The inside recovery

Speech

In the early weeks, I really feared that I would never be able to converse easily and that I would progressively forget more words than I could remember. It is the most frustrating incapacity to suffer and those who have any more of it than I do have my sincerest sympathy.

I developed this fear before I sloughed off the "jargon talk" habit, that is during the first three or four weeks of recovery. In that period everything was a bit of a mystery and I didn't know what I didn't know. But I knew enough about word-finding to bother me.

Several times I have resolved to keep a little notebook with me. I would write down words that I had found after I or someone else had found them for me. Then any time I forgot a word I could look to see if it was one I had lost before but then found again.

Sleeps and moods

My tendency to sleep late in the morning is no less pronounced now than it was while I was in the N&N and in Caroline House. I developed a liking for a 20-minute power nap at almost any time during the day; it works to give a noticeable boost of energy.

There have been plenty of times when I have felt that the effort needed to get through the next mission was just too much; missions like buying new clothes, selling the old flat or going back to the optician, again and again, to get the glasses to fit properly. Maybe I sometimes got downhearted but not — I claim — self-pitying.

How do I feel about the experience now? Given the circumstances, I feel pretty good and can present a cheery face to the world. Daily living is less of a burden and "missions" hold less dread. And now I keep busy meeting people and doing things I had never dreamed of.

During these weeks

This is the tally of what more I could do in each of these weeks:

1   Fluent aphasia (speaking jargon), pronounced, with a good littering of obscenities.
    Writing short lists of reminders (left handed).

2   Loss of speech fluency (possibly resulting from infection and antibiotics?).
    Able to follow simple instructions (like "watch my finger" and "eat your lunch").

3   Recovery of fluency of speech (still full o' jargon).
    Writing recollections of dreams and impressions of state of health (mainly jargon).

4   Starting to recognise own errors of speech.
    Difficulty learning names.
    Transition starts: from writing jargon to writing English.
    Transition ends: to writing English.
    Long sleeps continue; up to 14 hours at a stretch.

5   Errors of speech reducing: correction improving.
    Able to follow "difficult" instructions like those in tests
    the OT did with me.

6   In speech, difficulty with word-finding continues; not
    such a problem in writing.
    A few names easy to remember.

10 Getting better with all vocabulary when speaking.
    Fluency in writing almost normal.
    Long sleeps less frequent.

13 Writing right-handed resumed.

15 Speech sometimes disturbed — hesitant, even frightened
    into silence — if surprised or pressured (first weeks after
    rehab).

50 Speaking mostly normal but sometimes nervous and
    hesitant.

100 All speech and writing normal (so I say).

A note about a transcription

The Journal isn't all gibberish, just the beginning; if you have had a look you will already know this. But the early pages do set tricky puzzles for the reader … both before and after transcription.

This note is about A4 Sheet 2 (with footnote 14). Even as author I cannot interpret this page but I am intrigued by its sense of excitement. It is a short, two-paragraph essay, probably —

considering the extent of my self-absorption — a reflection on my own condition. There are several good-looking words and phrases hinting at subject matter: "many sleeps", "and awake but reflective", "writing", "Notise" (possibly as injunction: "Notice!").

Something not so obvious is a structure only partially revealed in the first paragraph. I clearly remember having a problem — when I was doing the writing — labelling a part of the text as "(a)" after I had used the label "(b)". Look towards the end of the first paragraph and find:

> ? a (b) a the 2 and 3 with …

The question mark and the letters "a" (one before and one after "b" in brackets) confirm my memory of the problem and my unfulfilled desire, then, to resolve it.

There ought to be an "a" in brackets, probably earlier in the text, but where is it? I think it is there, earlier in the paragraph as expected; find:

> it say to (a×t fen many sleeps …

It surely says, masked by untidy writing:

> it say to (a) Hen many sleeps …

or maybe:

> it say to (a) How many sleeps …

thus uncovering the mystery.

If you are a student of speech therapy or of linguistics may wish to work with more of the text. You are welcome to contact me via the Web site.

And finally …

There have been magic moments when I have achieved or felt some one thing for the first time. It's fun — at least for me — to see them all in one place. And I want to take the liberty of offering some advice.

Magic moments

These magic moments — lots of them — are roughly in calendar order; there must be others but these are the ones that stand out:

- Feeling the back of my neck. I had an itch and — without troubling myself — raised my right hand and scratched it. This was the first signal that strength was returning.

- Cutting food with a knife. I had been eating like an American for some weeks, left-handed, with a fork. The first time I used a knife right-handed was to score a banana at one end, so that I could peel it. (Actual cutting came a little later.)

- Standing up straight. It was a great feeling to be six feet tall again rather than sitting in a wheelchair. I still enjoy just standing and being tall.

- Standing upright to pee. It's a boy thing.

- Tying my laces. I was so pleased that I bragged about it to Jessica, my OT. She immediately made me do it three more times!

- Carrying a pear in a dish and walking at the same time. I wanted to save my pear for later but I was in the restaurant with my walking stick. I declined Rachel's offer to see me back to my room and walked all the way by myself.

- Blowing my nose with both hands.

- Feeling Nigel's arm across my shoulder. My sister and brother-in-law took me home for lunch at a time when I could only just transfer between wheelchair and car. Nigel acted as my prop to help me stagger into the house; I could feel the reach of his arm all the way across my back.

- Putting my watch on without thinking. During rehab I had a daily struggle to get my watch to balance on my left wrist while my weak, uncoördinated right hand tried to fasten the clip. One day it happened that I fastened the clip without realising; I had done it "on auto."

- Writing right-handed. The wrist-watch-fastening event inspired me the same day to try right-handed writing, and I could. (See Journal, 31 May.)

- Feeling my elbow touching my ribs. A big advance in sensitivity; the elbow felt the ribs and the ribs felt the elbow.

My advice to you, the survivor

We all know that every stroke patient has a different experience. You may be hardly affected or you may be laid up. My experience — "given the circumstances" as I like to remind myself — has been a fortunate one. Here are some reminders of how to make the best of your circumstances:

- Follow the advice from The Stroke Information Service: rest, take each day as it comes, don't cling to deadlines, keep to a manageable routine.

- Be ready for ups and downs. They can last for days, either way.

- Recognise your magic moments when they occur.

- Celebrate all your magic moments by telling everybody.

- Look forward to the next improvement even if you don't know what it will be, or when.

- Work hard; remember: the more you do, the more you can.

- Take other people's advice about seeking and accepting mechanical aids. Take your own advice about rejecting them … in time you'll be the stronger for it.

- Accept all the help you can get from family and friends; but do try not to be unnecessarily demanding!

If you haven't already read the Journal, have a go at it now. It was all written on the dates marked and provides a unique record from the inside of a patient. At the beginning it is a bit mysterious; once it gets going it is a mixture of the bland, the frank and the unexpected.

PART TWO
THE JOURNAL

About the Journal

This part of the book contains transcriptions from the various notes and the journal that I made during my stay in hospital and in rehabilitation. The transcription is as accurate as I could make it but you may think it still has errors. This is because there are errors in the original material and I have made no attempt to correct them.

Physical forms

I did the writing in three phases:

- The first few notes were made on a freebie, giveaway notepad; these individual A6 sheets are identified and the layout of the original handwritten material is roughly echoed by the transcription here.

- Next come the notes made on A4 unlined paper which my sister had brought for me the first week I was in the N&N; for these pages the layout of the handwriting is not followed.

- And finally the main journal was written in an A5 lined notebook.

Concerning dates

For the first few sheets dates are a bit unreliable. The days do not match up with dates, some dates were written for the day four days after the proper date (eg 21st for 17th) and sometimes the year was written as 2002 instead of 2004. It is convenient that the three writing media were used in the sequence described above; it means that it was easier to get the loose-leaf material into the right order.

Note that the loose-leaf and the notebook dates overlap during March and April.

Transcription and style

Some of the handwriting is truly illegible and it is shown by hash ('#') characters. Sometimes I have assumed a reading on the basis that most words, including the easily legible neologisms, follow English language conventions. There are few examples of unusual diphthongs or groups of consonants; I seem to have carried on writing by most of the rules of English. Based on this observation, I have made choices among doubtful readings which make words conform to those rules.

The early work shows a good grasp — with very few exceptions — of form: ie the conventions of text layout including indentation, paired parentheses, paired quotation marks, punctuation in general, and the uses of paragraphs and bullet points. This observation will be interesting for an academic analysis of the effects of the stroke — and the later recovery — when discussing the scattering of the components of intellectual functions among damaged and undamaged parts of the brain.

The Journal, March and April

Free notepad, 1 [1] [2]

Guelt advisor ta msg [3].
      re: visit at vinigt

- - - - - - - - - - - - - - - - - - -

Mary + Penny apoligies [4]
re: mail forg ton
      for nex forgahr
forget womet
      and collect
      com ne lt
upduirl, world
      conne to frodn
      correlt. Acco is to s
      cheo u resb ebrit

---

1   The layout of the texts on the first sheets is reflecting the handwriting as much as possible.

2   On the reverse of this sheet someone (possibly me) has later written "Possibly the first written note."

3   The abbreviation "msg" is for "message" and is reliable as a reading.

4   Mary and Penny were fellow students at the Norwich School of Art & Design.

67

Free notepad, 2

[name and address of insistent fellow patient]
— — — — — — — — — — — —

Mich [5] T'aI Chalin
Phone phone water
to say in with ad
T'ai Cugush

Free notepad, 3

Answer poor choice
    for meclna
All for the car while
    far far vilgit
    a bite as 2 [6] for
    a whotis.
40 Belod galled

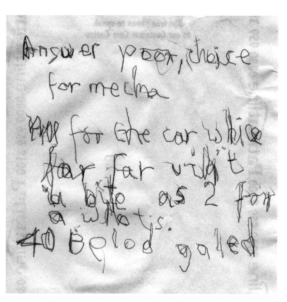

It is easier to decode the original hand writing than it is to decode this print-out. See that the numbers 2 and 40 are clear enough.

---

5   Could be Mike. my T'ai Chi Master

6   I am strongly of the opinion — even certain — that when I wrote Arabic numbers, they meant what they said. Two what and 40 what I cannot say.

Free notepad, 4

Dr Jetty Lotey [7]
Ring (Wells [8]) Caroline

— — — — — — — — — — —

Pho s and: massante
        at to surreands
        to msg for
        to msg to Welsh
Mike to the T'ai [9]
        Surroind texxxads

Free notepad, 5

My unsdider
        for the erished

---

7   Probably Dr Jenny Latoy, my GP at the time.

8   Wales, where my good friend Caroline lives. This looks like a
     reminder to make a phone call.

9   Mike Symonds, my T'ai Chi Master.

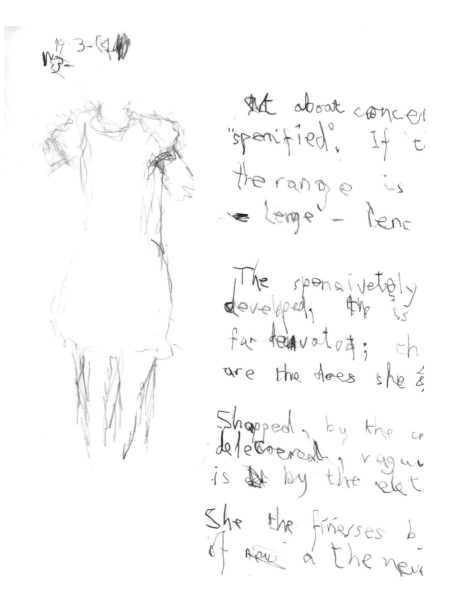

"Young Woman Dancing"
An essential element in the development, in a dream, of a theory of vision.

A4 sheet 1

19-3-04

~~Mt~~ aboat concerned "spenified". If the spe'c the range is regined
- lenge - lenc -lerm [10] [11]

The spensively is developed, the is for is far de~~x~~vatoot; thes there
are the does she ~~x~~ the noht.

Shapped, by the cropped, delecoereal, vaguuvely, be is ~~xx~~ by the
elethipirris

She the finesses by one of ~~xxx~~ a the never these - next - the fine
foured the, next never she courntry four nexet, vatceguue ~~x~~ velue
and the hengfed and and will where word any forgiven.

---

10   The first two paragraphs describe a theory of vision; the last
     two denounce the theory in no uncertain terms. The theory is
     illustrated by the young woman dancing. My excited exploration
     of the theory came after seeing the young woman in a dream:
     at each moment the dancer in the dream is expressing a new
     movement of the head and limbs or a new costume. The same
     sequence starts again viewing her from a slightly different
     position in space. The theory was that the brain stores all the
     possible images of the dancer and recognises what is actually
     happening by matching the true, seen dancer with one of the
     images in the brain's mental library. Hmm, nonsense! And so the
     last two paragraphs vigorously expound the counterarguments.

11   The sequence "- lenge - lenc -lerm" matches the speech pattern
     of muttering, experimentally, looking for the right word. (See
     Commentary.) Considering the spacing of the dashes, we might
     take it that I was trying to write an aside — a bit like this — that
     was not completed. See also 28th March.

A4 sheet 2

Suggusigittifity! High fightfy fairfully! It's it is it it it it say it say say have it say to (axt fen many sleeps a ad# awake - but reflective [13] - with the rx (at on for from brought a brake) from it is 2 or 3 roloan is or cle an as [14] ? a (b) a the 2 and 3 with hare - zoxogh galiblantail; the taplatslip by writing is in writing is haverter.

Notise with guesseg auting (with for of galaing) xx with clocking turning turning, the durning matharn I thosing to chosen then x twicks twicks out twice. The "burning" on genefulk if #that is at the that of a quicking: doing so is a out a a xxxxxxxxx gisaliot (?). A agaiat is not a rairing and wrilling a with nirtllay on a logging a to ## #####

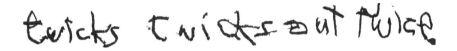

---

12   Date written in a different hand.

13   Hyphen at line break.

14   Right from the start this page brings a sense of excitement. It seems to be an assessment of how I am.

Structure in the first paragraph is partially revealed by the letter "b" in brackets. It is not entirely clear what other part of the text is wanting the label "(a)". See *A note about a transcription* at the end of *What happened next* for a possible answer to the puzzle.

A4 sheet 3

Wed 22th March. [15]

(Hopt the is a ꭓif out)
(the adtoan adw are)

March curve courve courve to kend
     and spare can,

Mars kye is at a taker for to
     repearet of freedoms to cermatorny
     with with & certermony rec#mony
                  say ret#apat#

---

15   22nd March was a Monday.

A4 sheet 4 [16]

Whendney 23 (o … ie 3rd of 3rd follow dasigh).

1. Charyth: the right rightfly right on sole you and improgafal if improvaxemadoylay. Aolay on on but a vere is is is is stregthen and a latactact & roughnnenneining

2. These right row raironmess- [17]
   - Chowraisp, partitral 1 + 2 thurmail & 5 load film [18]
   - Chaim   OK to to pail up nurnes (noses only)
   - Chaim clasesy to a glean new grenny to from from to from (from very wearkwhy read)

---

16   This sheet is the first to have a clear tie-up with the theme that was central to the following writings, namely the patient's assessment of his own condition.

17   Here follows a short catalogue of conditions.

18   The numbers 1, 2 and 5 refer to my thumb, index finger and little finger ("load film" = "little finger"?), the only ones that had any movement, just a few millimetres each.

A4 sheet 5

Monday 23 (a) [19] I to a sketch from of [20]

I to war 2 from from from:

-- to gaw way about below flow & flow are but flow was 2 flow
form 2 from.

fail to

revecy

to at   (is sight froa

top of   but about

picture [see diagram overleaf]   inloss frow)

a sceping

scrapering

camang

(dropping show showping correc to edge)

-- to was to way arraraga#l#yallary:
to emptininway can a way collect it the enteffihesions with
shelgnegs shell on tow.

---

19   This sheet claims to be a Monday sheet (a) as if there is a sheet (b);
     indeed there is: it is A4 sheet 6.

20   This page also attempted to record a dream. In the dream, I had
     seen a view of a jar of ready-made mayonnaise or, possibly, one or
     another brand of instant coffee (their jars are similar shapes). The
     view was of the jar seen very close up so that the top of the jar was
     above the line of sight and the bottom well below. In addition, the
     rendition of the view was as a line drawing which rendered the
     label on the jar transparent so that all the details could be seen
     through the labels and the glass, without distortion. The sketches
     were a part of the explanation, but not very successful; the vision
     had been somewhat in the style of Japanese manga animated
     films.

monday 23 (a)   I to a sketh from of

I to was 2 from from from:
= to saw way about below flow flow flow are
but flow was 2 flow form 2 from,

faird to
reveal
to of
top of
picture.

(is right from
but about
inless frow)

a sceping
scrapering
(amaro
dropping show showping correg to age)
= to was to sway arraroga flgalars:

to emptinin way can a way collect
it the ent of thesions with shelo hass
shell en on too.

A4 sheet 5: the sketch of the screw-topped glass jar is surrounded by
explanatory notes but it doesn't do justice to the dream's vision.

76

A4 sheet 6

Mangay 23 (b)

A4 sheet 7 [21]

Mar 28 (Mar 24th) [22]

Even an as see charge.
Envet I turn never till till turner.

-----//-----

This morning - one neartming - morh warm on 1 day 1 day 1
days as checq'c chalom'chs chormons' chormen's [23]. Next next
to next mark!

A4 sheet 8 [24]

Tuesday 20th April 2004

1. Very bright morning.

2. We started our upper body programme.

3. Probably three pieces of writing is enough.

---

21 This was intended to be a page of aphorisms (!).

22 Date corrected by my son Roger; this is the last page before my
move to Caroline House on Thursday 25th March.

23 See how the word, with its apostrophe-S, has been tried four
different ways.

24 (Last of the A4 sheets.) Several attempts during mid and late April
at right handwriting practice including this quite neat sheet. It
was the last successful attempt until the end of May.

The A5 Notebook starts

The first pages are individually identified but from the beginning of April — four weeks from the stroke — the journal entries are transcribed without regard to pages; each entry is dated. Up till the beginning of April, all was written in pencil; after that it was in ball point pen.

Page 1

Note at front
(27 Mar - last of 3 monday)

See addrus at back
(This note as yesterday)

REMIND: THING NOTES

Page 2

23   Pleare remard to remard toate's toothe & elethromoloque likewith reqblickard (aned) [25]

Mybe nigh for nightot's confrete … but the confisetert has certairnly easier the system's formattered.

----

* Monday (ie 1 mudkey = Monday)
        (~~south~~ last of month) [26]

Ganfivere the giverned. I will will do a little more hand writting.

----

* Query: 29 March [27]

Page 3

Visual field:

1.   Left field, reflorted format favaoured by few not disgravated imageves.

2. a.   Left images, focus.

   b.   Blurred are returned; x will try arresting.

See natured accordion next.

---

25   This looks like a reminder to ask family to bring electric toothbrush.

26   If this means the last day of the month (rather than the last Monday) that would have been Wednesday 31 March.

27   In ball point pen, likely on a different date.

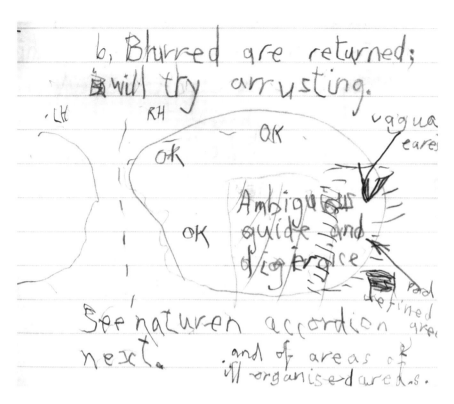

6, Blurred are returned;
will try arrusting.

·LH   RH
            ok
        ok   OK   vagua
                                              eare
                Ambiguous
            ok guide and
                difference
                                            refined
                                               are
    See naturen accordion
    next.   and of areas of
            ill organised areas.

The "RH" eye's diagram in support of the text on Page 3 and Page 4.
The "LH" eye is ignored because it has no problems.

81

Page 4

(View of right as site.) [28]

-- The "plot" has reguires are very & where horis and very edges.

-- The xxxxx xxxxx x to left left-handed his indberd, firt edged

-- The outboard edges lost differend x

-- The edge is m#stly poorly defened by ended vaqueness - see sketch (not done)

---

28   Refer again to the diagrams in the Commentary (*In the first few weeks*) and on the previous page to understand the text. The area of blurred vision is very sharp edged at the top and inner margins and is vaguely defined towards the outside.

Page 5

Tuesday 30 Mar 2004

(Refers are easiers! You just look them in the ~~timer.~~ diarxy.) [29]

~~Also, mention error - I'm thank of tire ##### - to~~

Arhirists first by quick quificults.

Physio - Joni [30]

S. nurse - Liliath

Psychology - Jess

Auxially - Jill

Physio - Kath

Occupational Therapist - Jessica

Speech help (psych) - Simon

Page 6

Special ##erde - Dorothy

~~Phsyg.~~ Psych - Alison

Nurse - Isabel

---

29 From this day onwards, the dates are reliable because I am copying them out of the diary in my organiser.

30 A list of names made out at a time when I could not learn or remember any. Do not rely on this list.

Page 8 [31]

comade (sitting) ¿commode? [32]

urinal (standing)

amiodarone (sp)

Page 9

urine [33] FrI 2-Apr-20024

collect, via kidneys and urethrae, into bladder. When bladder full, content may release via the (male) penis. Body may standing, sitting or lying. Discharge of urine is nominally unrelated with rectal action.

Fecal material is dried and collected as it is moved to word's the (metres long) tube's end. Periodly the individdy voids it, for me please, before the busy starts.

---

31 Page 7 is blank.

32 This page and the next, plus some that are interpolated later, were written at a time when I was not sure my body was working correctly.

33 At this period, I was convinced — in a delirium kind of way — that my body was not working properly; and in a small way it wasn't: constipation had set in. I wrote what I thought was a logical description of what should happen, as a way of reassuring myself. The feeling stayed but the body kept working.

Dated entries, April

Sat 3-Apr-2004 (April = mth 4) [34]

There seem to have been no recordable dream activity. During the first weeks, there were plenty of nightmare. Over the last 10 - 8 days the nightmares seem to have disappeared … dreams too … leaving an apparently dream desert (!) for a whole week.

Tired today. Greater range of flexible, range and strength in right arm. Aiming [35], of course, is a risk undertaking (both for the (for weapon and for target). [36] [37]

---

34 From this point entries are identified by date rather than page-number.

35 This refers to any attempt to use the right hand.

36 This example of a writing-competence error has two parts to its explanation: in the first place the left hand hides what it has just written; the short term memory failure explains the doubling of the left-hand part of the bracketed expression.

37 The weapon being the hand and the target whatever I was trying to grasp or carry.

Tue 6-Ap-20024

After a day off it seems that the writing is gradually settling into a # style. [38] "Gradually" maybe a bit optimistic; there are many old habits to automate: do all/some letters adopt clockwise/anticlockwise … does letter-spacing settle down … does production speed up … in fact "gradually" will be a bit of a dream while practise [39] continues.

More activity in the class-room: dressing & washing. It's surprising how much you do: partly from learning how to do things and partly from working harder doing the new jobs. Must remember to keep glasses to hand; for me, even putting on a sweatshirk [40] is 8 times easier when I can see what I'm doing.

Wed 7-Apr-2004

Busy day, lot's [41] of work (including importune right hand) but I did feel in need a long rest between sessions.

Although this journal is just fine for keeping notes, larger of flat pieces of paper will do a better for p#ctising "calligraphy".

---

38 All this refers to being left-handed writer.

39 "Practice" noun, "practise" verb … you choose. Normally I would have written "practising."

40 Please remember that I have tried most accurately to transcribe the original material.

41 Erroneous apostrophe.

Thur 8.Apr-2002

First night in new room a bit wild in terms of sleep. The neighbour's tv had its sound turned up well beyond a normal bed time even to $1^{\underline{00}}$. ($1^{\circ}/_{c}$).

Room a great success: light and airy, lots of space and view the over the garden on two sides.

Maddy has quite rightly said that I should be making specific notes on my advances. This day my speciality has been in the hands.

Just before dawn I fell an itch would be satisfied if I could scratch the back of the scalp - neckline, midline. So I scratched the back of my neck - with my right hand. [42]

Strong physio session with hand work; while standing (!) and with use of left hand "forbidden". [43]

---

42   It doesn't sound much but it was a life-changing experience.

43   This is the incident of turning the pages of a glossy magazine.

Fri 9-Apr-2004 (Good Friday)

Not such a good day: feeling most of the day as would rather spend it in bed, and recover from that sense of "sleep to rebuild".

My handwriting took a knock! it was the first outing with the right hand! About half an hour - many of whose minutes were re-picking-up the last pen - taken to write a few words and make two (?3?) pictures (see file). Rather pleased, considering the mood I was in. [44]

Did sort out wardrobe; must learn and practice [45] letter "W".

Handwriting faster; I am relying on practice more than on careful technique to build speed and style.

Sat 10-Apr-2004

As yesterday, so today: feeling in need of "sleep to rebuild". Generally peeky, but not actually ill.

Good visit - and not too short - from Maddy, Natalie & Flossie. Had them all in fits about trying to moisten my figure with a lick when I wanted to the page of a magazine. All the while standing at a desk and holding my <u>left</u> hand behind my desk. [46] (Ie: in physio last Thurs.)

---

44 Moody? Yes … the folder with my earliest writings had gone missing three or four days earlier. (It was found, see 11 April.)

45 As before.

46 … behind my back.

Sun 11-Apr-2004

The good news is that the lost notes have been found. [47] I had the idea of asking a small-handed visitor - i.e. Flossie - to look behind the drawer with the hidden section [48]. Several hands came together to take the drawer ... and there was the lost file. It was the last possible and it paid off.

Of course, I am very pleased indeed. [49]

Lovely visit from family, the presents and flowers (I have a stash of olives). Tim tuned the tv to all 5 channels. Flossie installed a birdfeefer, Maddy brought much appreciated and shamefully played down laundrey. And Nigel is undertaking the production of some personal stationery.

Right hand stronger - a bit - a unwieldi; lots, but showing willing!

---

47   While I was in the first room, I was making my notes on the A4 stationery with the pencils that Maddy had brought for me. I kept them in a folder — a plastic slip-in folder — and they went missing. I did not suspect theft but I did suspect accidental throwing-away; it was a sad loss for me because these notes contained the first writing I had done and I regarded them as very important. I was moody about the subject right up the day that the notes were found.

48   The little chest of drawers on wheels came with me when I moved rooms and so this search became possible.

49   The "notes" referred to are those very early attempts at keeping a journal written on the A4 sheets. Their loss had made me particularly cross; had I accidentally thrown them away? had someone else? had someone treated them as rubbish? I was in tears at their recovery.

Mon 12-Apr-2004

Right foot can tap toe and heel ... can hear the difference but not feel it.

Right hand over-ambitious but must let it pace itself; I keep wanting it to do more.

Good ~~missing~~ visit from Maddy. Talked about she is, and everything is OK. Ate the amazing lamb sandwich (sp?) [50] ... too delicious for words.

Busy day tomorrow.

Tue 13-Apr-2004

Good sessions on a busy day. My hand did get tired and seemed to need a good rest.

Not such good news on the medical front: potential heart problems. Will be asking for a rerun of the explain as I didn't follow it all.

Even so, hand is more capable and flexible.   [51] has given me exercises - intl. [52] placistine (sp) - to do hand-strengthening.

---

50   Editing "on the fly"! Well, I think it's remarkable.

51   Blank space left for Therapy Assistant's name, forgotten at the time: June.

52   I think "intl." is an abbreviation for "international"; the so-called plasticine (*sic*) was an American product.

Wed 14-Apr-2004

Excellent review of medical situation from Dr. Louisa Ng. (Seems to be a risk of stroke or a risk oacclot - see description in file. [53])

Lots of physio - lots of work!

Thu 15-Apr-2004

Right-hand corner of mouth seems to be more sensitive.

Was v. tired this a.m. following a disturbed sleep. Better in mood and energy levels p.m. What a waste of energy it seems to note these tiny changes; but is actually useful and part of a progress/ assessment, and looms large in the consciousness so can hardly avoid being recorded.

The p.m. physio was to learn balancing while walking - eg: just lightly holding a rail with the left hand and being guided and protected on the other side.

Fr 16-Apr-2004

After the previous rough night's sleep and truly dozy morning, today was a revelation: sleep well, woke easily and "got up" with minimum hassle. Right arm feels as though it's been working hard but right fingers - in a quiet sounding and feeling place - can feel themselves. Eg fingertips distinct when touching the thumb one by one, and rubbing the fingertips - separately or together - with the fingertips clenched against the palm of the hand.

---

53 "file" refers to my collection of paperwork, and notes from staff. The comparison of risks is between a bleed (from blood thinning) and clot (from lack of thinning), either of which could trigger another stroke.

It has several times struck me - all the since that I came here - that there is a link with my very sleeps. Many times my body really wants a truly solid sleep; after the body has had such a hibernation (eg as much 13 - 14 hours) I feel as though the body's capability has taken - not gradual but measurable - a clear step forward. These massive sleeps have insistence over recent days though the improvements still came (most days).

Just now I told Joni about the sensitivities in my fingers, she asked me about the right leg … I can't truthfully say there is a clear focus (or locus) of sensation.

Today's physio advanced an extra step through the balancing and walking programme to include quad stick (note much easier in bare feet).

Sun 18-Apr-2004

A catch-up day for little things remembered.

I hadn't told Maddy that ever since ~~by~~ my Wash & Dry lesson [54] I had been standing - unsupervised - at the sink.

I hadn't discussed or written about eyesight for at least two weeks, could be three. In that time blind spots had disappeared (see note for Mon 29 Mar).

I hadn't put in anything about my rib. Slipt on left rib while picking up something. I guess an intercostal got snagged. It felt much worse today after sleeping on the left side. [55]

I hadn't said anything about feeling institutionalised. It came to

---

54   Correctly "Wash and Dress".

55   Doctor suggested pain-killers but I don't like too many inessential chemicals in my body.

me yesterday that I had become part of what goes on here. Of course I am, but perhaps too wholeheartedly. I need to continue bringing "self" to the flow and continue to bring my own ideas into play. (Such as tiny exercises for all parts of the body. [56])

Mon 19-Apr-2004

A disappointing day (possibly due to the cracked rib) having even yesterday and certainly today fallen below par: physical weaker, making several speech errors & lisps, and quite clearly under the weather. Diagnosis: cracked rib. Did OT & physio - just shorter sessions.

As last Friday, walked with no shoes & socks and trousers above the knees, for greatest visibility and sensitivity. Whereas FrI was done with full-length mirror, today was ~~particularly~~ partially with out mirrors. Total done with the quad stick: about 13 m.

Tue 20-Apr-2004

After today I got the real feeling of a day's work. The "U/B prog" is the upper body programme full of exercises for the upper body (!) So in this session I was writing right-handed [57], and learning strength exercises.

It was tough going and I finished tired. Part of the effort went into one of gym machine going for 5 mins each way, cycling then 5 mins each way on a quasi hand (foot) mill. Tired right-hand?

---

56 That's to say rather than just waiting to be told what to do and when.

57 Writing without convincing results.

Yes! Plus other elements of the "physio prog" <u>and</u> an exercise taking in loads of walking, with & without mirrors and with & without shoes, socks and visible knees. And finally the last 13m into my room, still using the quad stick (legs in civvies) and witnessed by Maddy - unknown to me - in suppressed excitement not having seen it before. Felt much better than Sun & Mon but not quite up to normal. Rib bruise obviously lessening.

Tues <u>last</u> week I remember as the day the pink blossoms started showing. Today we have double-pink flowers on the tree outside the window - halfway to a couple of bloom's work.[58]

Wed 21-Apr-2004

Having finished yesterday feeling like a labourer who did too much, I slept like a log and woke early, and still I felt I had done too much.

Good work with the walking: after one "run" with the quad-stake, I did some with a plain (adjustable) stick, some with bare feet again. I walked (frankly, with some help - tilting towards the weaker side a bit but) which was a great satisfaction. A even greater satisfaction came from 4 or 5 steps which I felt were very smooth in gait and rhythm.

Overall strength may well be going up in R.H. But feeling not particularly accurate: texture & weight not ready yet for using R.H. for eating, though I did use it with a knife (held as a pen) to neatly start the peeling of a banana at lunchtime.

---

58   A struggling joke on "double-pink flowers" and "a couple of bloom's-worth." And "bloom's-worth" should have been "blooms'-worth".

Other RH results in recent days include: blowing nose with both hands [59]; doing up laces (first report tomorrow [60]); making minor adjustment of wheelchair position using the RH wheel; "fast" action to un/lock the wheel; raising the height of the bedside table while still in bed. Thus it is that strengths collect.

There are plenty of jobs I won't try; many jobs that have to be done with the hand out of sight or that rely on the sense of texture. Hence the avoidance of wheelchair propulsion. [61]

Plenty of jobs can be done with the hand half out of sight; the other hand being the sight, and the job using the hand as a pair such as when getting dressed or dried.

Thu 22-Apr-2004

Finished the day feeling a bit washed out after the excitement.

Having bragged about tying my laces, Jessica (OT) had me showing how I did it - on and off the foot.

The big event was having Nigel, Maddy & me having lessons & practice getting in & out the car. And going for a drive. The road trip was definitely a bit overwhelming and I flopped for a real sleep this afternoon.

---

59 This was a long-held ambition. Among the many ways of dividing the world's population into two parts, one must be the ability to blow one's nose single-handed or the inability. I belong to the latter group.

60 I remember reporting this to Jessica to which she immediately replied "Show me"! So my OT put me through a trial, three times, proving that I could do what I said I could.

61 This (propulsion) in contrast to making minor adjustments of the location of the wheelchair.

Sun 25-Apr-2004

(Family meeting all went fine [62])

Was un peu disappointed by RH progress. Not justified, considering the achievements I listed only last Weds and the little tricks that accumulate daily.

Excellent car trip with M & N in and around the city, the patch where I feel overall the most comfortable.

I believe that as I am writing slowly <u>and</u> beyond the last 3 - 4 letters I can't read what I've written, so it quite often changes what (longer) word I write or even starts a new phrase, (as well as other kinds of error).

Mon 26-Apr-2004

There is a change in the atmosphere as RHP the patient turns into RHP the rehabilitator. The emphasis is on "why" as much as "how". Eg walking is taught as "how", of course, but as much for the reason of going anywhere, and so be taught the (old) techniques you need again.

Likewise, the true uses of all the handcrafts such as you need in every room in the house.

The basic training is still the greatest amount of work, the advanced training takes increased increasing emphasis.

(Old leather diary has full list of activities.)

---

62   The Family Meeting being a colloquium of staff, the patient and the patient's family, to discuss the situation and what will be happening next.

Wed 28-Apr-2004

Tired today even after good sleeps. Mon & Tues busy; still can overdo things.

Trying more RH writing; v. poor advances.

Maddy came with a couple of books and announced that she has diabetes. It is and will be a shock both to the daily (treatment) and long-term (diet & weight) living. [63]

Fri 30-Apr-2004

The end of a disappointing week, full of hope and so off-colour and lacking energy.

Spoke to Dr. Agreed it was nothing serious, possibly trying too hard, possibly frustrated by the lack of wished-for progress.

In the p.m. three lady visitors Penny & Mary have called several times always full of cheer and giving a delightful sense of being with pals chatting.

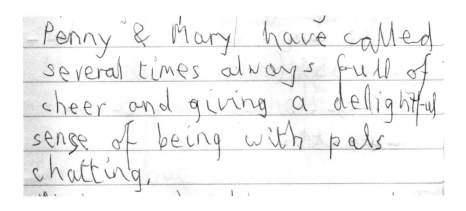

---

63   A false alarm, I'm happy to report.

Nairne, who lives round the corner, came having recovered from (?) kidney troubles. News about NCAS and the King Street festival.

Realised how long it is reporting on RH sensitivities: heel (tiny bit); spot/itch on neck; eyebrow (50%); nostril, ear rim and a greater proportion of the scalp; arm - wrist to shoulder - about 15% (on an arbitrary scale) … anything to do with the sock? [64]

---

64   Elasticated tubular bandage worn all the way up the right arm.

The month of May

Tue 4-May-2004

Visits and visitors at the weekend. On Sat p.m. Maddy collected me just before 4 and we met Nigel & Flossie at 4 by the little turn-in for the Castle. Back to theirs for a coffee & chat. Great outing, and got back after an overlap with Cynny up for the w/end. [65]

Sun - sunny - Cyn visit & tour of all the gardens on the site and unexpected visit by Tess whom I hadn't seen for months. Cyn lives in London but Tess only lives round the corner so I might see the latter the sooner.

Mon - rainy - Cyn visit and drive home. No school today as it's May Day.

Wed 5-May-2004

The fingers on my RH have noticeably swollen over the last week or so. Seems to be about "drainage" and "fluids" and is not unusual for stroke cases. Massage towards the heart and rest with the hand in the air (eg on a cushion). Coincidence or certainty? The RH is busier and stronger.

---

65   Cynny is my sister living in London.

FrI 7-May-2004

Had a go with a PC y'day. All is/will be OK. RH good for slow typing; LH good for mouse and, presumably, for pen + tablet.

I wonder why the transfer to LH has been so relatively easy. Maybe it's because the RH is (currently) so slow. I'm on the verge of giving up RH writing and concentrateding on strength and general utility.

Test on RH forearm revealed sensitivity to touch on the thumb side and little-finger side and - on thumb - the angle it set (ie by therapist): open, halfway or closed.

Wed 12-May-2004

Even since last FrI there have been noticeable changes on RHS; including: toe to scalp sensitivity to touch; sole of foot kind of ticklish; stronger arm & hand as evidenced by frequent, low-speed of use to propel wheelchair, and holding knife for eating.

Walking with stick in room unsupervised, the length of the corridor supervised (~ 30 m).

Had, s/wich & coffee lunch with Jennie Cunningham at the Forum, then recital at the Assembly House. First time I've felt normal, and not the least bit tired.

Thurs 13-May-2004

Did walking today, out of (33) room, across lawn and up path to benches * which back on the ring road, down to fish pond * and then back to room the quick way [66]. * With suitable rests!

RH foot & hand given experimental very cold stimuli. Wrist to elbow respond with "Ow, ow" and hand hardly noticed the chill. Can't say anything definite about the foot. [67]

Tue 18-May-2004

So much can happen in just a few days, in particular in the walking department. Almost all my locomotion - in the daytime - is by foot, with stick. At the ends of the day I used the w/chair to guard against errors of the sleepiness or fatigue. I say "used" because now I've been moved into the flat (little studio flat) [68] with the w/chair parked outside in the corridor (at Joni's direction!). All locomotion is by foot and very careful.

Had proper Orme lunch on Sunday and sat out in the garden.[69]

This p.m. a trip out to the Sainsbury Centre with O.T. Jessica.

---

66   The quick way was directly from the garden to the outside door of my room; it would have taken a much longer walk to come through the building.

67   I had been to a presentation by two physio students who had each spent four weeks at the hospital. In their talk they had referred to the sharing of one of the nerve pathways by nerves for temperature and for pain. Joni's experiment on me vividly showed how the sensations could cross over!

68   On the previous day, Monday 18th.

69   This remark apparently out of place; probably refers to Sunday 16th.

Sun 23-May-2004

What a tough week! 8 physio sessions plus, plus lots of activities. Even after a quiet Saturday I'm still shaky in all departments (including writing).

It's clear that I need to build up balance and stamina, and that will take a long time. I'm really quite down in the dumps with fatigue. This week schedule is lighter, thank goodness.

Mon 31-May-2004; Bank Holiday

It took most of last week to cheer up - helped by feeling stronger and by having two offers of (commercially let) a ground flat [70].

Also good progress on all fronts esp. RH which is both stronger and cleverer so that, for example, cooking on Thursday was a lot easier and this morning I put my watch on without noticing.

[71] It took most of last week to cheer up - helped by feeling stronger and by having two offers of (commercially let) a ground floor flat [72].

Also good progress on all fronts esp. RH which is both stronger and cleverer so that, for example, cooking on Thursday was a lot easier and this morning I put my watch on without noticing, and then I tried writing ... seems to be OK! [73]

---

70 Properly: "ground floor flat."

71 From this point, writing was with the right hand; the first attempts being this paragraph and the next as a copy of the previous two. (With minor correction, made subconsciously.)

72 This is the subconscious correction.

73 It was the happy accident of noticing that I had put my watch on without noticing that was my inspiration to try writing right handed.

I must say that I am fully chuffed by being able to write, however scratchily. But it is better than the unnatural-feeling lumpy left. Obviously it'll take a few days to be normal - or maybe weeks. And another thing…

The Month of June

Tues 1-Jun-2004

... RH doesn't get neglected so often; it's much more reliable - just over the last week - holding and carrying things, eg bits of clothing, papers, book or - as today - a bowl with a pear in it, from the canteen to the flat, while walking with stick. I suspect that this has as much to do with strength i'th'arm as strict neglect. [74]

Appointment to view flat in Wood Street confirmed for Friday a.m.

This is writing with a thin-bodied pen, (ball point). Neater?

This is writing with a thick-bodied pen (ball point). Smaller?

I notice that all the writing skills came back together; not just the letter shapes but little habits such as completing the letter 'i' with its dot before moving on to the next letter

| About taste buds |
| About the flat |

(also crossing 't's.). I also noticed that a lot of writing makes your hand tired, up to the elbow. [75]

---

[74] No! "neglect" has a proper technical meaning and I was using it incorrectly here. Instead of "strict neglect" I should have said "not paying attention to where the arm is." My OT described it as "... Richard's ® arm which he does tend to leave behind on occasions."

[75] The notes "About" were to remind me of subjects I should record.

Sun 6-Jun2004

Saw flat in Wood St on Fri. Maddy & Nigel - and Jessica & Evelyn as advisors. All on one level, access at rear so easy parking for electric buggy. Paid deposit.

left hand: When I first came here, nothing really tasted right or smelled right. Savoury things had sharp overtones of an unsuccessful curry; sweet thing (eg fruit, eg puddings) were more successful; strongly and characteristically flavoured food and drink (including wine, both instant & real coffee and plain choc as examples), these all lacked true flavour as if the bottle, jar or packet had be [76] hotted up and left open for 3 months before using.

In the last 3 - 4 weeks, the background flavour went, the aromas came more nearly true. The neutral taste in ~~may~~ my empty mouth was more like the blood from a bite or a tooth [77]. If the unsuccessful curry taste were characterised as yellow then the empty mouth would be pink. The mouth has become almost neutral in the same 3 - 4 week period.

I'm giving RH as much work and responsibility as it can take. It is limited by strength, stamina and touch! - but it's coming along fine.

---

76   … had been …

77   Eg when brushing too vigorously.

Sun 13-June-2004

This past week has been interesting [78] in that it had strong similarities with the weeks I was first here: long, strong sleeps - with vivid dreams - and daily improvements in performance. These improvements are both from the body's own recovery and from the physio and O.T. strengthening: RHS skin - top to toe - feels itches, surely a sign of nerve paths reconnecting; walking is more even, to the extent that I have found myself setting off - out of my room - without the stick (always without a walking stick within the room); much improved balance, I can stand on RH foot for several seconds; eating RH with spoon (eg for cereals & puddings) as well as with knife; increasing impatience - living in hospital - ready to go home! [79]

[End of the first 100 days] [80]

I just saw a young blackbird hopping across the grass; it missed its footing and fell over sideways. Most comical. [81]

---

78   After being moved out of The Flat on Monday 7th into a regular single room.

79   Went home 21 June.

80   This is just how I wrote it: larger and in square brackets.

81   The spirit of Sei Shōnagon was upon me.

Recipes

(At the other end of the A5 notebook is a note of the Occupational Therapy cooking sessions., spelling errors included.)

Lunches what I made

— Open ham & tomato sandwich with green salad.

— Cowboy's breakfast (baked beans on bacon on toast)

— Fried Haloumi cheese with hot tomato sauce and cous cous. (onion, tinned tomatoes, herbs, Tabasco)

— Ratatuile + baked potato, topped with grilled cheese

— Garlic mushrooms finished with white wine & cream, and spaghetti

— Cod filet (3 mins µwave), mushroom sauce (using crème fraiche) & new potatos

ORGANISATIONS AND INFORMATION SOURCES

Different Strokes

Highly regarded source of valuable, practical information as well as support for the "invisible" emotional side of life.

http://www.differentstrokes.co.uk/

The following is quoted directly from their Web site as at December, 2005:

"Different Strokes is a registered charity providing a unique, free service to younger stroke survivors throughout the United Kingdom. Our services and the number of stroke survivors benefiting from them have grown dramatically since we were formed in 1996. We are run by stroke survivors for stroke survivors, for active self help and mutual support. "

9 Canon Harnett Court
Wolverton Mill
Milton Keynes
MK12 5NF

Helpline: 0845 130 7172

The Stroke Association

Probably the better known organisation, The Stroke Association is both another solid source of information and "The Stroke Association's main focus is to support people who have had a stroke and their families. We do this by providing **information** and **community services**." (Quoted from Web site, December 2005.)

http://www.stroke.org.uk/

Stroke Information Service
The Stroke Association
240 City Road
London
EC1V 2PR

Helpline: 0845 3033 100

Other associations

Most parts of the country have stroke associations or clubs. Some are affiliated to the national The Stroke Association. You can find yours in different ways such as through the Internet and from flyers pinned up in your GP's waiting room or at your rehab centre.

The Internet

With only the simplest guesswork you can get relevant information off the Internet. I freely use Google and succeed with searches such as:

- For support organisations: "stroke association mycounty" (put your own county name in); and "carer support".

- For background and technical medical information, just choose a small selection of words as in: "CT MRI scan", "fluent aphasia" and "stroke ischemic"

You can confine your searches to Britain by adding this to the end of your Web search: "site:.uk" (without the quote marks); or select the button "pages from the UK".